ELISABETH BING'S GUIDE TO MOVING THROUGH PREGNANCY

Other books by Elisabeth Bing

Six Practical Lessons for an Easier Childbirth
Having a Baby After 30 *(with Libby Colman)*
Making Love During Pregnancy *(with Libby Colman)*

ELISABETH BING'S GUIDE TO MOVING THROUGH PREGNANCY

With a foreword by Sheila Kitzinger

Photographs by Jill Strickman

The Noonday Press

Farrar, Straus and Giroux · New York

To Peter

Copyright © 1991 by Elisabeth Bing
All rights reserved
Foreword copyright © 1991 by Sheila Kitzinger
Photographs copyright © 1991 by Jill Strickman
Photo retouching by Fred Marshall
Designed by Jacqueline Schuman
Published simultaneously in Canada by HarperCollins*CanadaLtd*
Printed in the United States of America

Library of Congress Cataloging-in-Publication Data
Bing, Elisabeth D.
    [Guide to moving through pregnancy]
    Elisabeth Bing's guide to moving through pregnancy : advice from
America's foremost childbirth educator on making pregnancy as
physically comfortable as possible at home and at work / with a
foreword by Sheila Kitzinger ; photographs by Jill Strickman.
        p.   cm.
    1. Pregnancy—Popular works.   2. Exercise for women—Popular
works.   I. Title.   II. Title: Guide to moving through pregnancy.
    RG525.B542   1991   618.2'4—dc20   91-21457 CIP

An earlier book on the same subject by the author, *Moving Through Pregnancy*,
was published in 1975 by Bobbs-Merrill

CONTENTS

FOREWORD

Birth is movement. It is the movement of a child burrowing and turning in the depths of a woman's body, pressing through the gradually unfolding tissues of her perineum, down into light, air, and space, and up into the safe haven of her welcoming arms. It is the movement of the mother's pelvis as she breathes deep into its resonating cave and rocks, tilts, and swings it in great circles to help her baby slide down to emerge from the confines of her body. In a harmonious environment, and among loving helpers, where a woman is free to move spontaneously, birth often becomes a passionate dance.

It is sad that much of the assistance that is offered by professionals in modern hospitals tends to impede and interfere with that movement. Today women are striving to explore and to respect the inherent rhythms of birth and to rediscover its spontaneous movements.

Pregnancy is movement, too. When a woman walks,

she rocks her baby up and down in the cradle of her pelvis. With each complete breath in and out, her diaphragm presses down, her rib cage swings out, her abdominal wall swells up, and breaths flow through her body in swelling waves.

Shakespeare described a woman with child as like a ship in full sail. A pregnant woman who moves well, with inner confidence and vitality, is often very beautiful. She bears witness to life in the ripeness of her body.

Yet to possess this grace, this fullness, she needs to feel positive about the changes that pregnancy has produced in her body. She needs to know how to move without strain, with economy of muscular effort, and in a way that acknowledges and celebrates her new center of balance—the heavy, melon-smooth curve of her belly.

In this book Elisabeth Bing shows how a woman can move in pregnancy so as to avoid physical stress and to enhance her sense of well-being. As she moves, she tones her muscles and prepares herself for birth in a way that, because it is unforced and harmonious, enables her to become more aware of her body. This helps her work with her body in childbirth, instead of fighting it or trying to close herself off from the intense sensations of her contractions and the movement of her baby toward her life.

After the baby is born, a woman's sense of well-being is intimately bound with the way she moves and carries her body, too. Once full, she is now empty. Her breasts are orbs of richness swelling with milk for her baby, yet they are also exquisitely tender. Because a standard part of a Western way of birth is a deliberate, and usually unnecessary, surgical wounding of the mother in an episiotomy, her vagina is raw and throbbing, and stitches may pull on sensitive tissue. Her body feels so different, so alien, that she may fear that she will never be able to express herself through it with pleasurable spontaneity again.

She needs to get back in touch with her body, to get to know it in this changed new form, and to feel that she is in control of it. That, too, involves movement: first, gentle movements of her abdominal wall and pelvis; then movements in which she explores how her pelvic floor muscles can squeeze gently and release, then hug tight and release, until she has these important muscles well toned and can actually "smile" with them, and smile generously and often through any ordinary day.

That is at the center of what Elisabeth Bing is teaching. Exercises are best taken out of exercise sessions and incorporated into our daily lives, so that they become part of the way we sit and stand and move.

Through all the events of pregnancy, birth, and the weeks afterward, movement is at the heart of a woman's well-being, and a vital element in her self-confidence as she starts out on the new adventure of motherhood.

—Sheila Kitzinger

ELISABETH BING'S GUIDE TO MOVING THROUGH PREGNANCY

INTRODUCTION

My own insecurity and lack of knowledge during pregnancy led me, almost twenty years ago, to write my first book on making pregnancy physically comfortable. I wanted to find out how women could move through pregnancy as gracefully and as energetically as possible, and how they could cope with everyday chores without hurting the baby or themselves. Much has changed, but I believe women still have the same kinds of concerns during pregnancy, many of which I hope this book will alleviate.

I have watched women for decades and worked with them throughout the childbearing years. Today, the professional woman knows how difficult it is to fulfill all her roles, in her career as well as in her home. This makes it even harder for her to accept the fact that her whole life-style will change when she has a child. As a result, she often seems to deny her pregnancy and to pretend that she is too busy even to think about her expected baby and her constantly changing body. Even her regular visits to her doctor seem secondary during her pregnancy. The many taboos that doctors today impose, such as no cigarettes, very little coffee or tea, no cold medications, no alcohol, not even the occasional glass of wine, won't make her concentrate on the baby she is carrying.

It may seem as if today's women have lost the ability to enjoy their pregnancy. Have they given up making room for the expected child? I don't really think so. The expectant mother may have lost some of the excitement of her pregnancy, but she certainly makes up for it once the baby is born.

Our assumptions about exercise have certainly changed in the last few decades. Someone said to me years ago: "Exercising, now that I'm pregnant? I'm sure it can't be safe. And, anyway, I never exercised much even before I was pregnant." Today everyone exercises, everyone is very aware of the benefits of keeping in good health and in shape, and everyone believes that a healthy routine should be followed in pregnancy.

Many years ago, Dr. Alan Guttmacher, a recognized authority in the obstetrical field, told the following story to one of my classes: "One of my clients was an acrobatic dancer. I had been looking after her for several months, when she arrived one morning with two tickets in her hands, saying, 'These are for you and your wife. My husband and I are performing next Saturday at the Palladium, and we would like you to come.' I was so intrigued to see a woman well into her eighth month of pregnancy dance that I went. I must admit I was worried. After all, I was responsible for her well-being and the child she was going to give birth to. When the curtain rose, she appeared in a long, loose, flowing gown and began to move, at first, quite sedately. Soon the music changed, became faster and more energetic. She was thrown high in the air, caught by her husband, and continued her dance. "I could not believe my eyes," said Dr. Guttmacher. "She was perfectly at ease and able to perform the most intricate movements and jumps without any harm to herself and her baby."

Dr. Guttmacher's experience, although unusual, no longer seems unique. Exercise and childbirth classes have become a normal part of prenatal care. Yet both the caregiver, the obstetrician or midwife, and the pregnant woman are more concerned today about the safety of the baby. This seems a dichotomy. On the one hand, you can do whatever you want; on the other, there are more taboos for the pregnant woman than there were ten years ago. How safe is safe? When can exercise be started, at what point should it be discontinued? I don't think there is a definitive answer to these questions, and obviously every woman and every pregnancy should be considered individually.

An obstetrician once told me about a discussion he had with an equally prominent colleague about what exercises they permitted their pregnant patients and where they drew the line. To their astonishment, they realized that each of them forbade the sport they themselves hated most, but were perfectly willing to allow women to pursue the sports they loved.

I feel very confident about trusting a woman's awareness of her limitations late in pregnancy. The woman in her third trimester will find that she will automatically slow down. She will feel the added weight of her baby; she will get tired more easily. Her heart will have to pump considerably harder to distribute blood, the volume of which is increased during pregnancy by about 40 to 50 percent. If there are clinical reasons to restrict her activities, her care-giver will certainly advise her. Otherwise, I think a woman should be encouraged to move well, as it will make her feel better and less clumsy.

I still remember the excitement I felt during my own pregnancy. I realized how little I knew about how much my body would change and what adjustments I would have to make. Theoretically, every woman knows that her body will change radically during these nine months, but I think it is just as difficult now as it was for me so many years ago to accept all the changes.

The first trimester did not cause many difficulties. My belly hardly showed. In fact, I liked to push it out more, just so people could see that I was expecting a child. But in the first few weeks I realized that I was easily tired and that it took me longer than usual to recover from fatigue.

Also, I was a little worried. Was it safe to run around at my usual pace? Should I still run after a bus to try and catch it? What about carrying heavy packages? In short, could I go on leading a normal life as if there were no extraordinary changes going on in my body?

I soon found out that I could do anything I normally did. In fact, my doctor encouraged me to stay active. But the tiredness persisted throughout the first trimester. I found it a good policy not to let fatigue build up, as it seemed to take much longer than usual to get my energy back. I learned to listen to my body. It was not always easy to take ten minutes off and put my feet up, but whenever possible, I gave my body the rest it asked for.

I cheerfully grew into my second trimester. I was not

nearly as tired anymore; I did not fall asleep everywhere I went! I also had to get maternity clothes, and there was no doubt anymore that my waistline had disappeared and that people thought I had put on quite a lot of weight. Those were the people who did not know I was pregnant. My friends cheered me on, telling me about their own experiences. They often seemed to live with me and my changing body. I felt full of energy and thought it would be great to be pregnant forever.

There were other surprises, which nobody had mentioned to me and which I had not come across in the many books I had devoured. Lovemaking seemed more fun. My husband and I felt almost liberated now that we didn't have to worry about whether I would get pregnant. My genital organs seemed to be more sensitive, due to the increased blood circulation. We had a wonderful time making love with great abandon. My size did not bother us; in fact, my larger breasts and their greater sensitivity seemed to please my husband, and he loved the roundness of my belly. Since then I have written a book on the subject: *Making Love During Pregnancy*.

I know that many women have difficulty maintaining a positive self-image when their bodies change so radically. They frequently wonder how they can still be desirable. I tell women that artists in every century have admired the pregnant body. Beautiful paintings and sculptures from ancient Greece to modern times attest to that. Our "different bodies" are only temporary, and it is intriguing to watch the growth of the fetus, to observe its movements, and to realize a little further on that the tightening of the abdominal muscles is a contraction of the uterus. Some women feel that tightening more than others. It is good to realize that the uterus is practicing for the day when the baby will be fully formed and the uterus can go into action to help the birth.

By my third trimester, moving about had become a little more difficult. It was easiest to let my husband help with certain activities, such as pulling on my boots. I decided to take Lamaze childbirth classes. I had been teaching them for a number of years myself, but to my great surprise, I was not a bit bored. I met a number of other couples who were at about the same stage of pregnancy as I was then, about the end of the seventh month. It was wonderful to share with my fellow students anxieties, aches, pains, joys, and great anticipation. Apparently an expert in the field, I asked the same kinds of questions I had previously answered in my role as instructor!

To illustrate both the timeless and the new problems today's pregnant woman confronts, I have chosen Mary, who is thirty-five and expecting her second child. Mary has studied numerous books and articles on pregnancy. They tell her what changes to make in her life-style in the next few months, what diet to follow, how much to rest, how much to exercise, and how to avoid anxieties, but she does not really see *herself* in any of this. Her common sense tells her that her daily routine can't change completely because she is pregnant.

Pregnant women need a program that fits into an active life, not the one outlined in the usual pregnancy article that seems to be directed at a fantasy woman who bears little resemblance to her real-life counterpart. In describing Mary, I am giving the active, involved, committed woman an exercise program, or really a "nonexercise" program, which she can incorporate into her busy schedule. This is certainly not a now-we-are-doing-our-prenatal-exercise manual, but it is a book that will help all women who want to incorporate healthy movement into their full schedules without having to set aside specific hours or half hours each day for "exercising." I also give those who prefer an exercise routine the chance to follow such a regimen. The photographs of a day in Mary's life offer an easy guide to use every day, from early pregnancy to the beginning of labor. All the exercises in this book are meant to be adjusted to your own personal comfort and ability.

Mary is pregnant with her second child, unlike most of the readers of this book. However, I do frequently have one or two couples in my childbirth classes who are expecting their second child. They often decide not only to take a refresher session but to participate in the whole course again.

"Last time we were expecting a child, it was an entirely new experience," one couple said. "We were tremendously excited throughout the pregnancy. It seemed an absolutely unique event for us. This time, we have hardly had time to concentrate on the pregnancy. Our older daughter needs a great deal of nurturing, we work, and suddenly we find ourselves only two months away from the birth of our second child, and we've had so little time to prepare. To be quite honest, it does not seem nearly as exciting as it was the first time around."

This is a normal approach to a second child. Obviously, the high measure of excitement and awe cannot be repeated, but a new sense of security prevails: the knowledge that you can cope with labor and delivery, and also that several years of parenting experience will make the arrival of the new baby easier.

I describe an average week in Mary's life to show how easy it is to incorporate exercises into an ordinary day. Mary is in her eighth month of pregnancy, but all through the previous seven months she has been following a healthy routine. By this time, the weight of her unborn child hardly bothers her during her normal activities. But even the very active woman finds certain movements tiresome as she increases in size. Little things like managing to get her stockings on when a large belly is in the way, tying shoes, or even getting out of bed can become big things if she doesn't know how to do them properly. Normally, one never thinks of these routine actions as posing problems, and it frequently comes as a surprise to women that they need to ask their partner's help. In the pages that follow, I have tried to give the prospective mother tips that will make all these tasks much easier.

I hope this book will help you use your body correctly and with the least amount of strain and, just as important, will help you enjoy your pregnancy.

PREGNANCY AT HOME

MORNING

Who would ever think that getting out of bed could be difficult? That is, if you don't count the great problem of waking up, becoming sufficiently conscious, and achieving enough willpower to swing your legs out of bed and sleepily start another day. But just physically getting out of bed when you are encumbered with a big belly becomes a challenge, a challenge that increases as the size of your belly increases.

The alarm has rung, you feel stiff, sleepy, angry, and even more awkward than usual because of the difficulty of sitting up straight over a big abdomen.

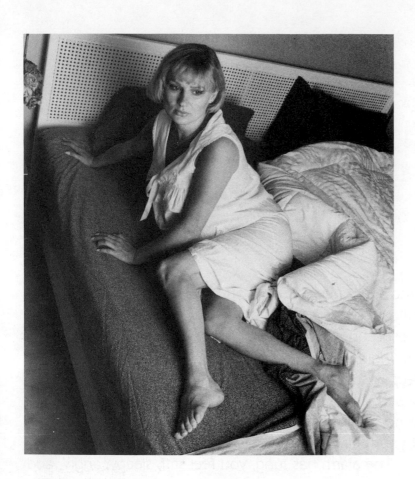

Sitting Up in Bed

Try this: Bend your legs, roll over on one side, push yourself up with your hands, and sit upright. After a night's rest, it will feel good to help your circulation increase by rotating your feet. Many women get leg cramps when they first wake up, or they may get them in the middle of the night and be woken up by painful cramps in the calf muscles. This is generally caused by stretching your toes, legs, and arms while you are still in a lying position. It may also be caused by a maldistribution of calcium in your body during pregnancy. Avoid stretching your feet and toes to get rid of the cramps.

Feet Exercise

Remember to sit up right away, now bend your feet up toward you and gently stretch your legs. Then, with your feet flexed or bent toward you, rotate them first out, then down, in and up, reverse down, out and up. Repeat the rotation three to four times. All this won't take more than two minutes, if that.

Here is an alternative way to get rid of leg cramps, a remedy which I learned in China: the moment the cramp occurs, squeeze your upper lip with your index finger and thumb, hold on for a few minutes, and the cramp will disappear. This is acupressure, and I found that it works for almost everybody.

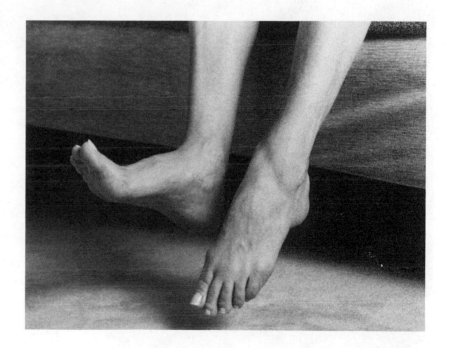

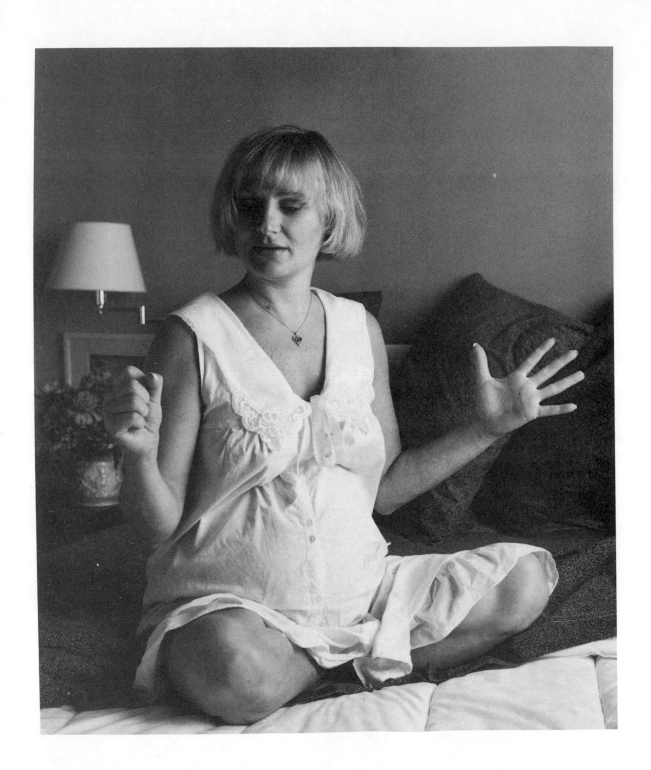

PREGNANCY AT HOME

Finger Exercise

Now sit cross-legged. Sitting "Indian-fashion" is good for you, as it stretches the pelvis bones and the pelvic muscles. Then bend your arms and give your fingers a workout. Make a fist, then stretch your fingers up and out, and repeat this at least four or five times. Frequently, one's fingers feel stiff and even swollen upon waking up. This is generally due to fluid retention, which occurs from time to time during pregnancy. You can help your circulation first thing in the morning with this easy finger exercise.

Getting Out of Bed

After exercising feet and fingers, it is much easier to get out of bed. Swing your legs over the side of the bed and stand up. It is important to follow instructions in the right order to make getting out of bed with a big belly as easy as possible.

Remember: Bend your legs.
Roll over to one side.
Push yourself up to a
sitting position with both hands.
Swing your legs over the side.
Stand up.

As you stand up, make it a habit to watch your posture. Stretch the top of your head and feel how your body aligns itself. It feels good to straighten up. You can actually be aware of carrying your baby with your own strong abdominal muscles.

Putting on Stockings

One of my students said to me the other day, "I can really do everything as I always could, but I seem to be slower and very often very clumsy." Perhaps some of my practical hints might make you less clumsy.

There are certain everyday routines which become slightly complicated when you are pregnant, and even something as prosaic as putting on stockings may suddenly seem to be a hurdle. It's difficult to try to lean or bend down to get close to your feet. And your partner may not always be available to help.

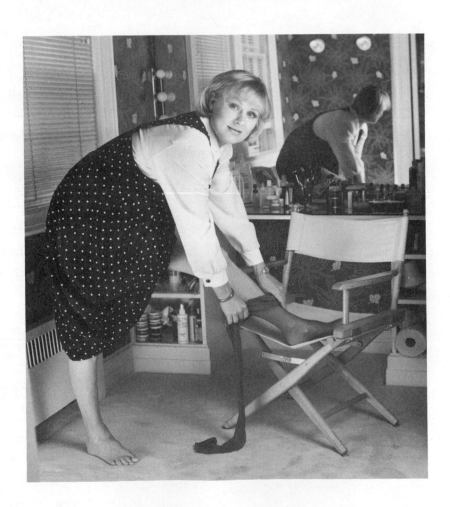

Try this: It's easier to bring one foot close to your arms. Look at the photo: Mary puts her right foot on a chair, which is slightly to the right of her. Then, as she bends toward her foot to put the stocking on, her big belly is as little in the way as possible, and she feels well supported by her standing leg on the chair. She straightens up as she pulls her stockings on.

Later in the book, I offer suggestions for putting on your shoes. (See page 34.)

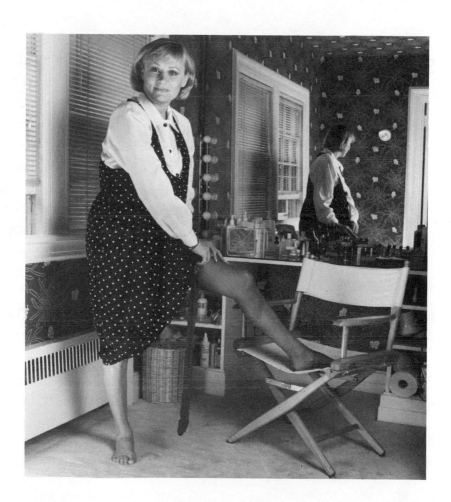

Stretching

Mary and Tom have a compact kitchen, the kind of kitchen you frequently find not only in big-city apartments but also in single-family houses in the suburbs or in smaller communities. Space is usually at a premium and everything is designed to fit with the least amount of waste.

Mary has to reach to get her cups and plates and saucers. Lifting your arms above your head and reaching up does not hurt you during pregnancy. A dreadful old wives' tale suggests that the baby may strangle on the cord if you stretch up. Strange women will come up to you in the supermarket and tell you to be careful. This is just superstition and nonsense. Stretching can't possibly do you or your baby any harm. The baby does not know that you are stretching up, though it may enjoy a little bit more space when you do, nor does the umbilical cord know it. In fact, it feels good to stretch and give yourself a little more space from time to time. So, if anybody comes along and tries to frighten you with such old stories, feel secure in the knowledge that you can raise your arms with impunity.

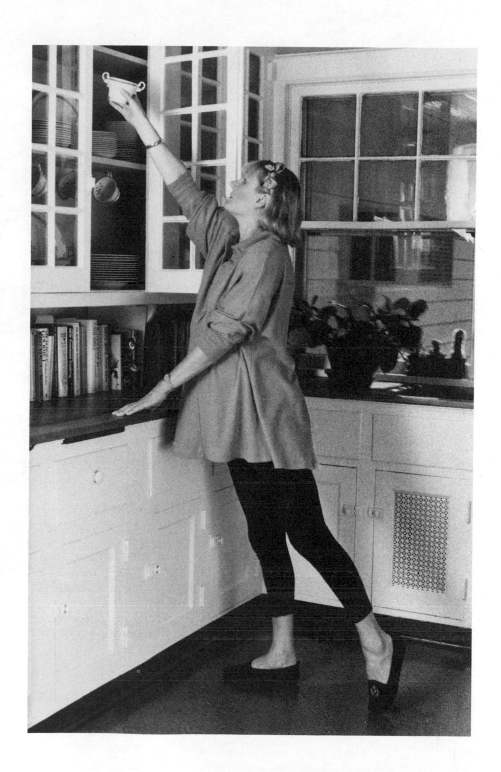

PREGNANCY AT HOME

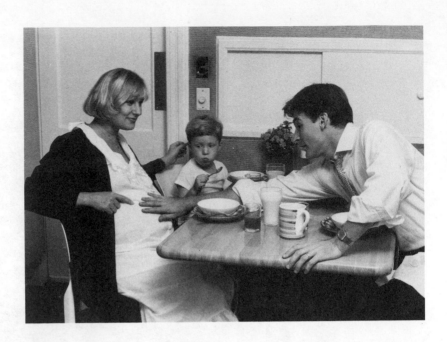

Breakfast

Breakfast is a fun meal. Tom has time to sit down with Mary and Matthew—though it is not every morning that they can all three be together for breakfast. Occasionally, Matthew has to be at his play group early, and Mary and a neighbor take turns taking the children to their group.

Mary looks wistfully at her plate and thinks that very soon there will be four of them at the breakfast table, and she wonders how she can get them all off to work, or play school, and eventually get herself off to work, too. But today there seems to be a little more time. It is a healthy breakfast. Cereal, which all three enjoy, coffee, fruit, a balanced but not fanatically healthy diet.

"Oh, look at the baby, it's kicking, it probably wants some breakfast!" says Tom and leans over and touches Mary's belly. "I can feel it move. Look, Matthew, see the baby moving. It's probably telling you that it wants to come out soon."

Resting

When you are pregnant, your heart has to pump harder with the increased blood supply. You will tire far more easily than in a nonpregnant state, and it takes longer to recover.

Few of us have the opportunity to rest a little after lunch. But it may be possible that even at work you can take fifteen to twenty minutes off, sit in a chair, and just slump, which means that you let your back sag, with your legs well apart, arms resting on your lap, head slightly falling forward, jaws and tongue relaxed.

Mary did not have a chance to take a break at the office. She takes the time at home. She lies down on her bed, knees bent, the upper knee in front of the lower one, and the knee and abdomen well supported by a pillow. This position relaxes the back, and the weight of the baby

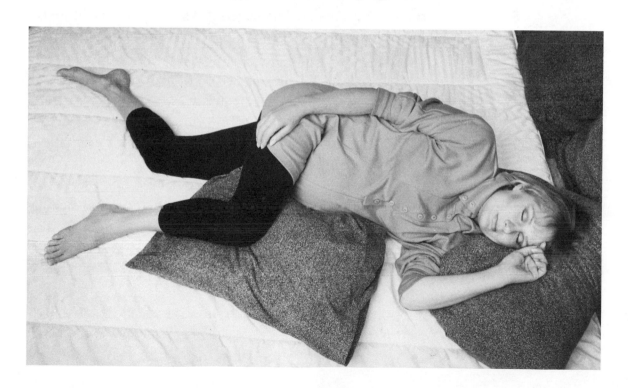

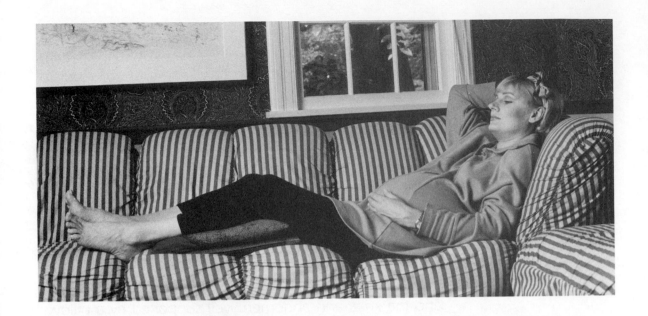

is carried by the bed. The baby is not lying on Mary's back, nor is it depressing Mary's main vein and artery. To lie on your back may be comfortable for a little while, but it is generally best to lie on your side when resting. The side position is often the most comfortable, but, as we are all built differently, you may have to find your own most comfortable position for resting or sleeping.

Occasionally, Mary can't find the time to lie down on the bed. She then lies on the floor for ten minutes, a pillow under her head and her legs resting on a chair. This will not only straighten her back but also relax her. By having her legs raised and supported on a chair, she aids the lymphatic flow in her legs. This helps to reduce any swelling she may have in her ankles.

In order to get up again, Mary rolls over to one side, supports herself with her arm and hand, and pushes herself up to a sitting position. This is the easiest way to get up without straining her abdominal muscles.

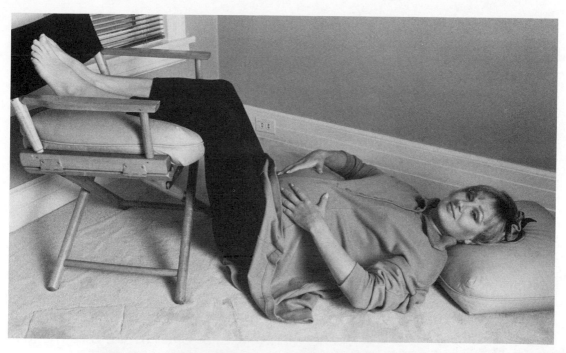

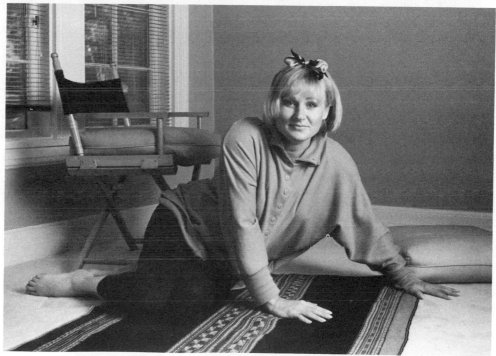

AT HOME—EARLY EVENING

You tire easily when you are pregnant. If you are still in your first trimester, I won't have to tell you how sleepy you are all the time, and how nice it would be to sleep practically around the clock. I remember my own pregnancy and my eternal sleepiness. I used to fall asleep at movies, theaters, concerts. My husband teased me and suggested that it might be cheaper to sleep at home.

It's not always easy to admit that you are tired. You feel fine, and for a great part of your pregnancy your ever-growing belly is hardly in your way. But tiredness comes on faster during these months than it usually would, and it takes at least twice as long to feel rested again. Therefore: whenever you can, sit down, rest, put your feet up, and stay comfortable for ten to fifteen minutes. Even if you don't have much time, try not to let fatigue accumulate.

At home, Mary relaxes as often as she can. The telephone rings, and she takes the call sitting on the floor cross-legged, leaning comfortably against the back of the sofa. During this short period before Mary has to prepare dinner, she takes the time to glance at the paper, or watch the evening news on television. At the same time, she exercises her legs, alternately sitting cross-legged or with legs apart, legs bending and stretching and so helping the circulation in them.

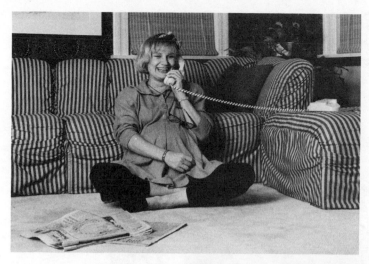

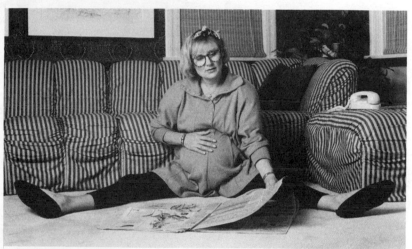

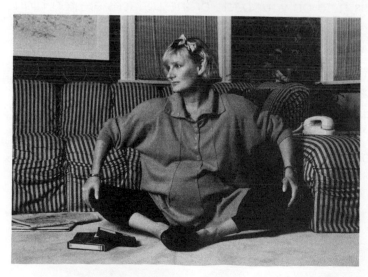

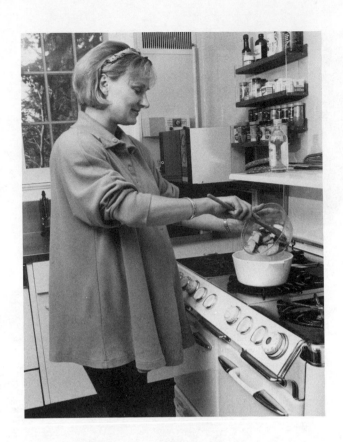

Preparing Dinner

I have found that most tabletops, sinks, stoves, and ironing boards are badly designed for the average woman, especially when she is pregnant. Depending, of course, on how tall you are you generally have to bend too far down, which is hard on your back, or the surfaces are too high or too deep. Whichever the problem, it's often backbreaking to work in the kitchen. With a big belly, it's difficult to reach across a table. When standing, you tend to hollow your back to reach forward. This posture overextends the back muscles and does not involve the abdominal muscles at all. It's therefore important to remember to stand straight, head pushed toward the ceiling, tail tucked in, and abdomen pulled up. You won't strain your back and you

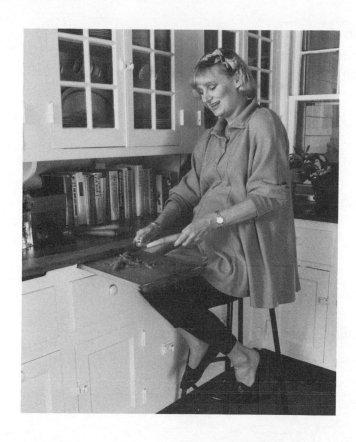

will support the baby well with your stomach muscles.

Mary looks relaxed and comfortable as she stirs the vegetables into the saucepan.

While Mary is preparing dinner and moving around in the kitchen, the baby seems very quiet. Perhaps he is asleep, as there is not much room to move when Mary uses her abdominal muscles. But the moment Mary sits down to rest, the baby decides to "go for a walk." Mary can actually see the movements of the baby, not just feel them. It is as if a wave is crossing her abdomen. Watching the baby move is exciting and reassuring, even if it is sometimes inconvenient to be kicked just when you want to rest.

Matthew's Bath

This is a fun time for Matthew, but it is also fun for Mary, because she and Matthew can play together before his bedtime. If they are lucky, Tom will be home before the bath is over and have a chance to enjoy splashing and laughter with his son.

But it can also be a strenuous time for Mary, because there is so much bending to be done. Mary remembers to use her body in such a way that there is little stress on her back. She places her legs well apart, feet firmly on the

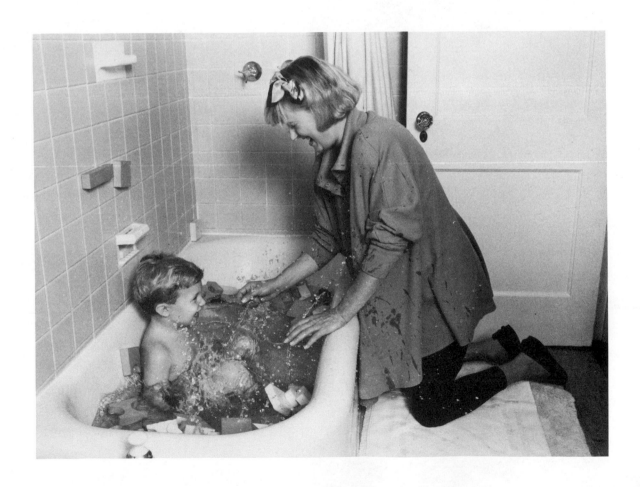

ground, then bends from her waist and keeps her back straight so that there is ample room for her belly. Mary is lucky that Matthew is tall enough to climb out of the tub by himself, and he only needs Mary to steady him. If your child is younger, it is even more important to use the position described above. But even that may become uncomfortable after a short time. Mary decides to lower herself by half kneeling and half squatting, so she does not have to stretch as far to reach Matthew or his many toys.

Tom walks in just in time to help Matthew out of the bath. Matthew is delighted to have both parents there to play with him.

Going to Bed

It has been a long day for Mary. She had to get up early to get breakfast for the family, to see that Matthew was ready to go to nursery school, to get dressed herself to get to the office on time. There was a great deal of work at the office, and even though she tried to rest between conferences and telephone calls, her work was tiring and it demanded all her attention.

At home again, late in the afternoon or early evening, Mary often has to read to Matthew or play with him, prepare dinner, and keep the house in some order.

I'm always amazed that women manage to function on all levels, particularly during pregnancy. Women work in an office, or wherever their profession takes them; they keep house; they look after a child; they exercise; they are companions and lovers for their husbands. In short, in spite of growing discomfort, they function well, even if they occasionally gripe about it all.

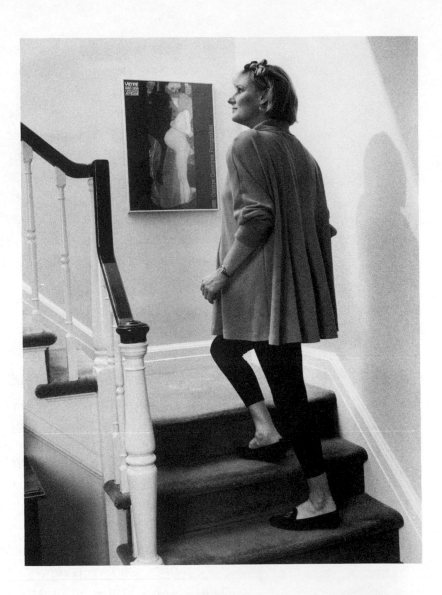

Climbing
the Stairs

But now it is time to go to bed. At this point, even climbing the one flight of stairs to the bedroom seems a fatiguing chore. Then Mary remembers what she has been told in her childbirth class: to manage stairs, straighten each knee at every step before lifting the other foot to climb the next step. This will slow you down a little, but at the same

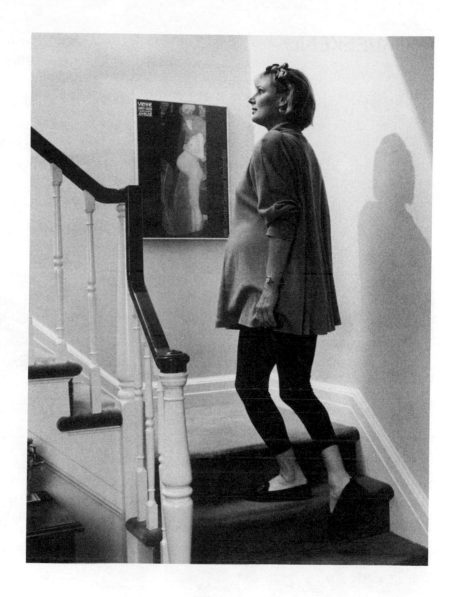

time it will distribute your weight well at each step and the pressure on your thighs will be far less. Usually—that is, in the nonpregnant state—we do not straighten one knee at each step, but keep both knees slightly bent. This puts a lot of pressure on the thighs.

THE WEEKEND

It's a beautiful day and Mary is ready to do some gardening. She is dressed for it, even wearing her new hat, which protects her from the sun.

Putting on shoes is not easy with a big belly in the way. The nicest thing would be to have Tom or someone else there to help give the extra tug to get them on. Alas, nobody is around to help at this moment. But Mary can manage by herself.

She sits on a bench and bends her left leg and rests it on her right thigh—that is, she brings her leg nearer to

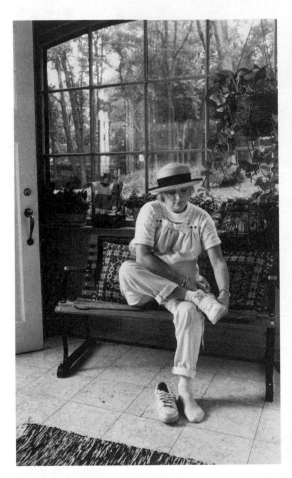
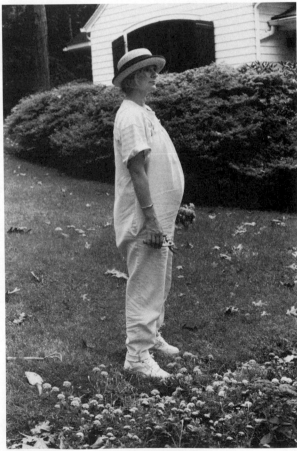

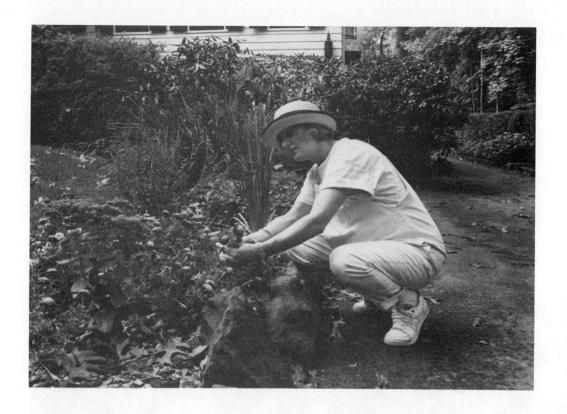

her arms. In this position, her belly is hardly in the way and she can easily reach the laces to tie her sneakers.

(Unlike Mary, put your shoes next to you, not on the floor.)

With garden scissors in hand, Mary looks to see which flowers she might cut to put in a vase. She is conscious of standing straight, her buttocks are tucked in, her shoulders are relaxed, and she is holding her baby up with her strong abdominal muscles. It feels very good to correct your posture from time to time, as it is far less tiring to use back and abdominal muscles to hold the baby up.

Mary squats down to pick flowers. She knows by now that, to pick up something, squatting is much easier than trying to bend over her big belly.

Grocery Shopping

The weekend is also the time to do the grocery shopping and the errands both Mary and Tom could not manage during the week while they were working.

Here is Mary carrying a bag of groceries in her arms.

Look at the first picture and see how she should <u>not</u> carry the heavy bag. Mary is holding the bag too high. In fact, she is supporting it with her abdomen. In order to do this, she is leaning back and overextending her back. This is likely to cause back strain and backache.

Look at the next picture. Mary is holding the groceries lower; she has straightened her back. If she is going only

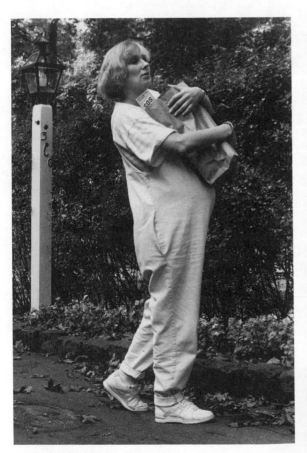
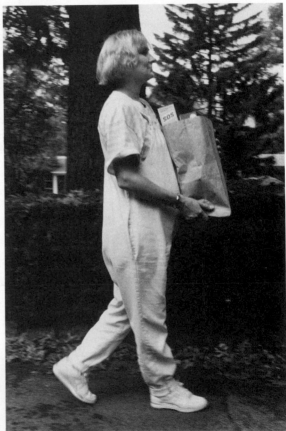

a short distance, she will be far less fatigued if she carries the bag with a straight back, using her arms to support the weight, instead of using her belly and straining her back. Mary is avoiding long walks while carrying heavy packages.

Before lunch, there may even be time to vacuum the house. Mary decides to consider this chore an exercise. She therefore quite consciously distributes her weight evenly on both legs, leans forward gently, and pushes the vacuum cleaner.

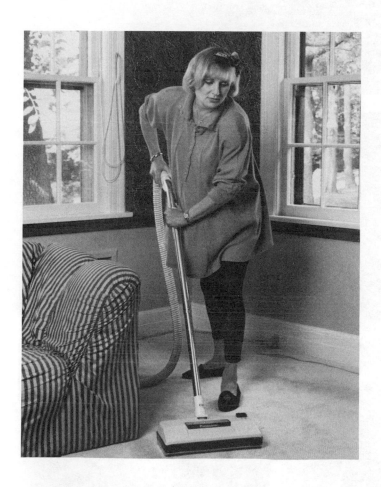

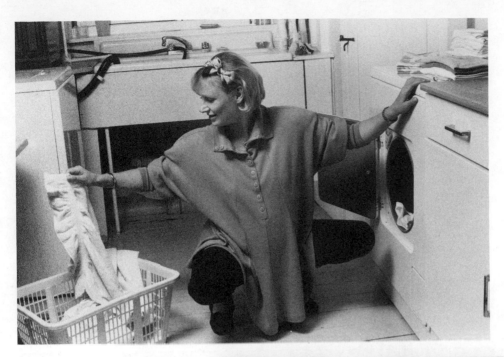

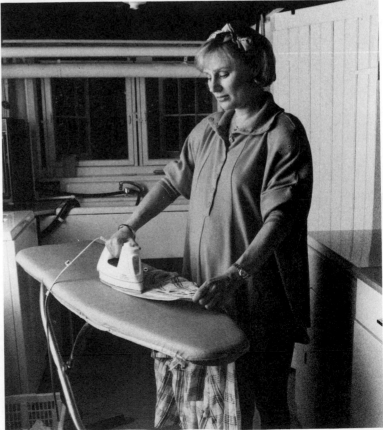

AFTERNOON

It is time for lunch. Tom helps to prepare it and Matthew helps to lay the table. After lunch, Mary will nap again to preserve her energy. She knows by now how important it is to rest as often as possible during the day and to take a nap if circumstances and time allow. She remembers how to get up from bed most easily. She rolls over to one side, and with her arms gently pushes herself up to a sitting position and then swings her legs over the side of the bed.

There are always more chores to be done, and Mary has a big basket of laundry waiting for her. To put the wash into the machine, she half kneels and half squats. Without having to bend over her belly, she can easily put the laundry into the washing machine.

If ironing has to be done, Mary has an ironing board which is at a good height for her so that she can stand straight and reach the board without having her belly too much in the way. You should not have to bend down over tables or ironing boards or raise your arms too high for comfort.

THE WHOLE
FAMILY EXERCISES

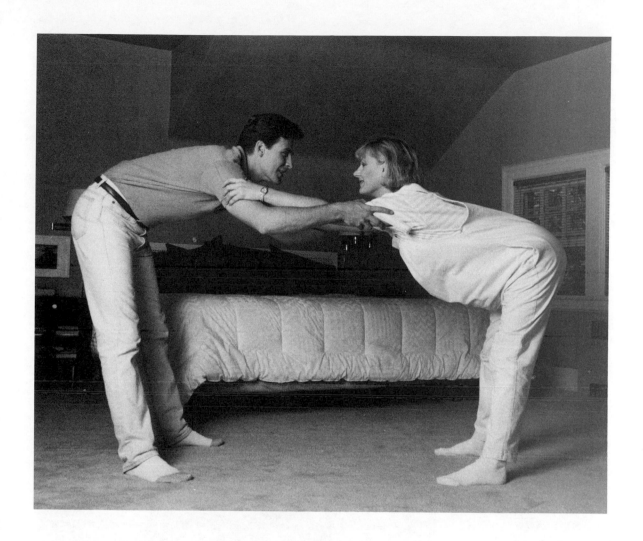

Spinal Stretch   Tom and Mary hold on to each other's arms and bend forward from their waists. Knees are straight and the head is raised. The legs are hip-width apart and the feet are parallel.

THE WHOLE FAMILY EXERCISES

Matthew always participates in his parents' exercise routine. He loves to work out with the grownups.

Back Exercise For Spinal Alignment

Tom, Mary, and Matthew start by standing upright. Mary watches her posture. She is holding her baby up with her strong abdominal muscles—shoulders relaxed and buttocks tucked in. All three inhale, and as they exhale, they slowly bend down, until their backs are so relaxed that they can touch the floor. Then, as they inhale again, they slowly straighten up, vertebra by vertebra, to a standing position.

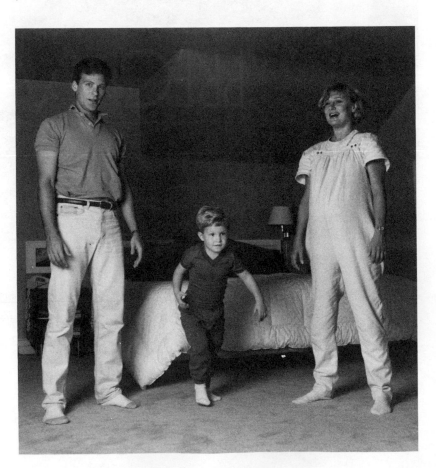

THE WHOLE FAMILY EXERCISES

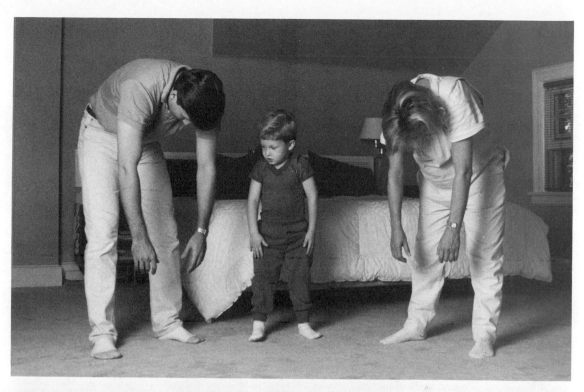

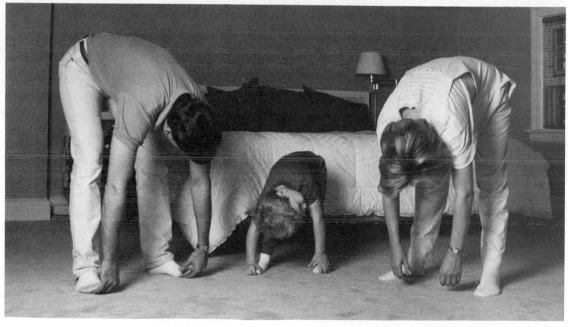

THE WHOLE FAMILY EXERCISES

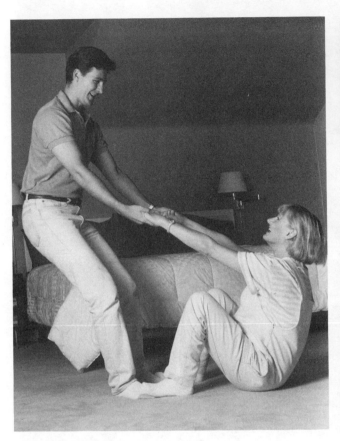

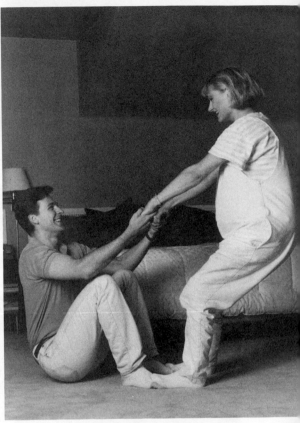

THE WHOLE FAMILY EXERCISES

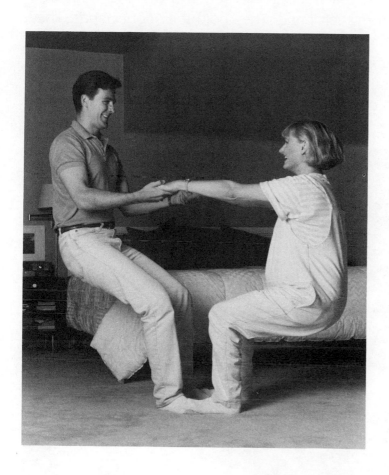

The Seesaw

Tom and Mary are standing close to each other. Mary rests her toes on Tom's feet. They hold hands and then alternately bend and straighten their legs, keeping their balance by supporting each other.

Side Stretch

Mary faces the camera. Tom faces the opposite direction. Tom's and Mary's right feet are placed against each other and Mary reaches with her left arm over her head and grips Tom's left hand. They hold their right hands. They inhale, and as they exhale, Mary reaches sideways, bending her left knee slightly. Then they reverse the movement, and as they exhale again, Mary bends to her left and gives Tom a good stretch to his left arm and side.

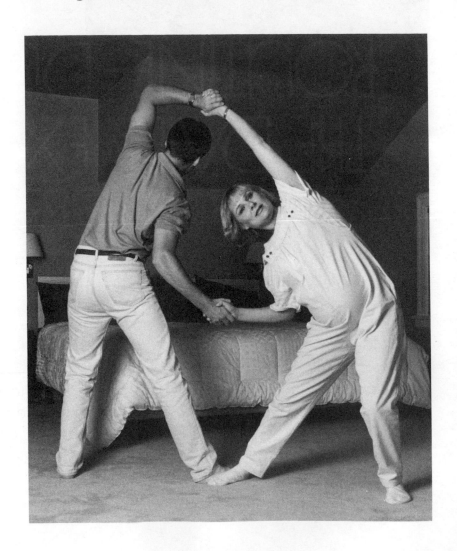

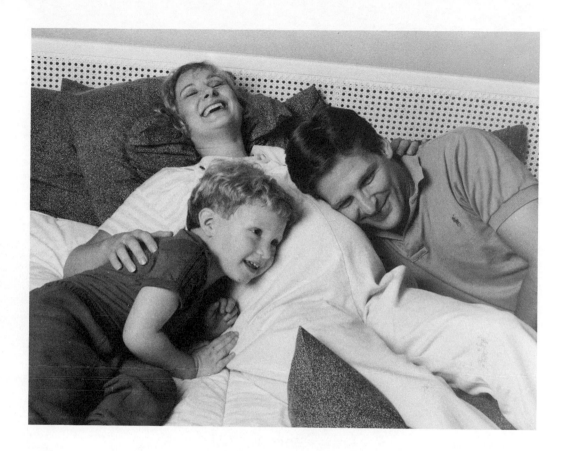

The family has finished exercising and Mary decides to lie down on the bed and relax. But the baby is kicking and rolling around. It could not move while Mary was exercising, so it is now trying to make up for the enforced rest. Both Tom and Matthew put their ears to Mary's belly to feel the baby move. They hope to hear the baby's heartbeat, but that is difficult with the naked ear. Toward the very end of Mary's pregnancy, Tom and Matthew may have a chance to hear the baby's heart, if Mary asks her doctor at her next visit to make a little pencil mark on her stomach at the place he found the heartbeat with his stethoscope.

PREGNANCY AT WORK

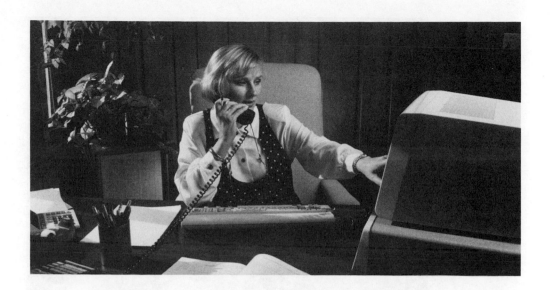

Mary wants to keep working as long as possible. It's a good feeling to get out of the house, to do one's own work. It is not always easy to be a mother and a professional woman at the same time, but Mary derives great satisfaction from her work. She enjoys her contact with the outside world, and she is quite sure that she is a better mother for working.

Of course, it is not every woman who can arrange to get back to work once she has a baby, or to arrange a leave of absence when she is expecting. Mary is lucky. Her office hours are flexible. As long as she manages the work required of her, no one seems to mind the exact hours she spends at the office.

Mary has found that it is essential for her to exercise during her working hours. She has a number of exercises that she can easily do in the office without interrupting her work or even having to get up.

Here are some of the exercises which Mary likes to do every day and which help her to feel good.

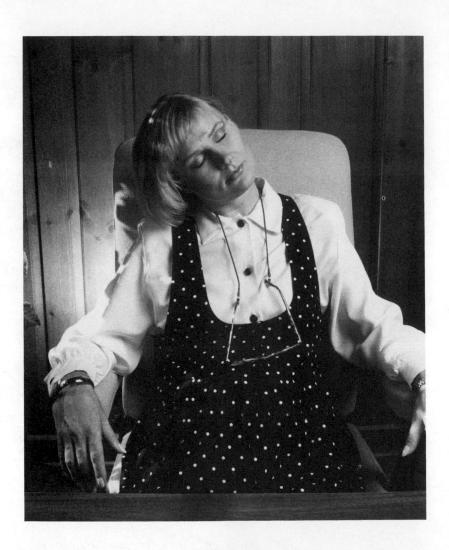

Head Rotation

Mary breathes in deeply and rotates her head to the right
and back. Then she exhales, rotates her head to the left
and forward again. She is careful not to raise her shoulders
as she rotates her head.

Shoulder and Upper Back Exercise

Mary breathes in and raises her arms forward to shoulder level, palms facing each other. She then rounds her upper back and lets her chin drop down as she inhales. Then she exhales and straightens her back again. She repeats this exercise five times.

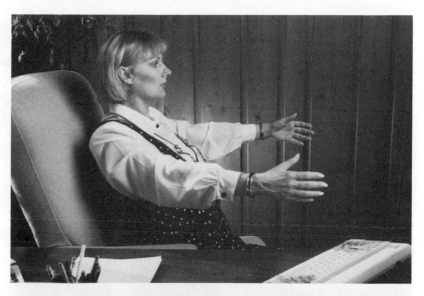

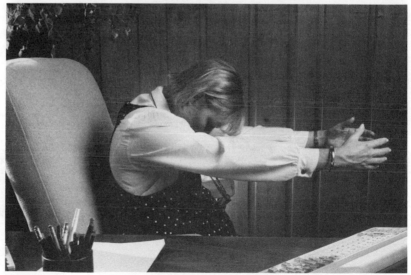

Shoulder Rotation

It feels good to stand up for a short while. Mary continues with a standing exercise, which, by the way, could also be easily done sitting. She stands very straight, then rotates her shoulders up, back, down, and forward. Mary repeats this exercise five times.

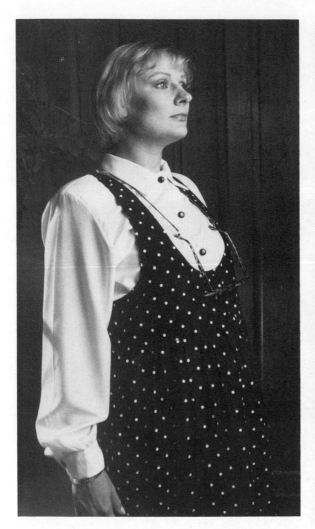 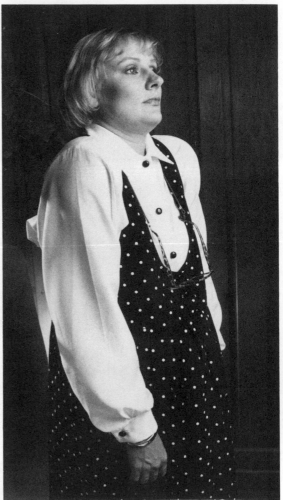

Side Stretch

Finally, Mary stands and lifts her right arm above her head and leans to the left, giving her right side a comfortable stretch. She then switches arms and does the same exercise with her left arm. Mary does this exercise five times to each side.

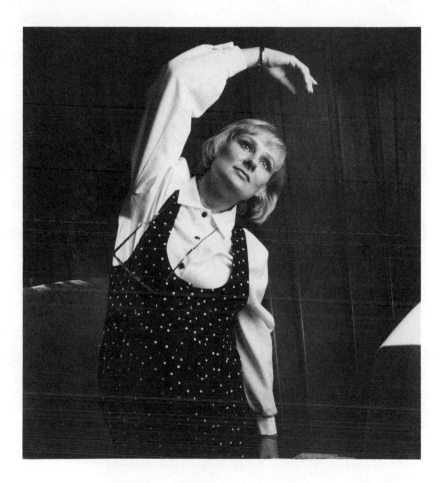

I am sure you can think of many more exercises sitting or standing. The ones shown here may inspire you and you can try out others without disturbing anyone or taking up too much space.

THE DAILY EXERCISE ROUTINE—DURING PREGNANCY

Try to go through this short list of exercises once a day. I realize that time might be at a premium, but do them as often as you can. You will feel better for exercising your body regularly. As your baby grows <u>in utero</u>, you will be very aware of pressures and muscle fatigue, backaches and occasional cramps. A regular routine will help alleviate most of those symptoms and annoyances.

The Kegel Exercises

There is one group of exercises which you should do every day, even without having a picture to remind you. These are the Kegel exercises, named after a California doctor, which help women develop strong pelvic floor muscles prenatally and also reeducate their pelvic floor muscle tone after the birth of the baby. These exercises can be done in any position, standing, sitting, or lying down. They can be done at any time during the day and whenever you remember to do them.

1. Tighten your front passage as if to stop yourself from urinating.
2. Tighten your vagina.
3. Finally, tighten your back passage as if to stop yourself from having a bowel movement. Hold everything tight for three to four seconds and release.

You should exercise your pelvic floor muscles at least twenty times a day. My gynecologist gave me an excellent tip when I complained how boring it was to do this series twenty times a day and how frequently I forgot to do them. He said, "Each time you urinate, stop the flow and let go again, and do this three or four times during urination." I got into the habit of doing this and found my ability to use my pelvic floor muscles greatly improved after some weeks.

Taking Exercise Classes vs. Renting Your Own Video

For myself, I prefer taking exercise classes. I like having company, and the camaraderie with other participants is important to me. However, some people prefer not to have an audience when they exercise, and it may be difficult to plan a busy schedule around an exercise class.

If you do take a class, find a teacher who is trained to give exercises to pregnant women and who also has a good knowledge of obstetrics. Exercises vary in difficulty from the first through the third trimester. But if you were exercising on a regular basis before you were pregnant, it is in all likelihood quite safe to do energetic exercises throughout your pregnancy. I am sure your doctor or midwife will give you advice as to the safety of strenuous exercises, including aerobics.

If you feel well, there is no reason to stop exercising at any point in your pregnancy. I find that most women know their own limitations well and do not overstrain themselves.

Hug and Lift the Baby

1. Sit upright, soles of feet together. Inhale, relax, and expand abdominal muscles, filling belly with air.
2. Exhale, contract abdominal muscles, hugging and lifting the baby.

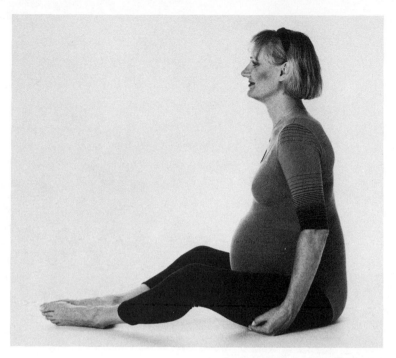

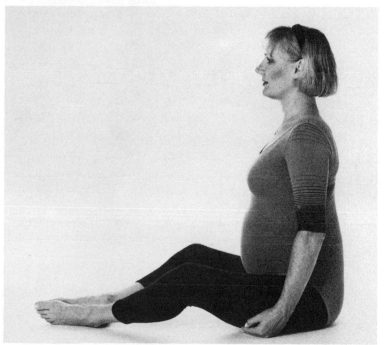

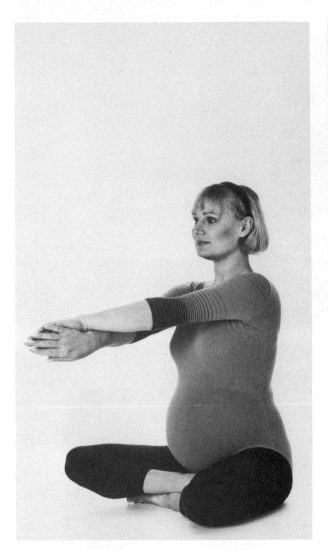
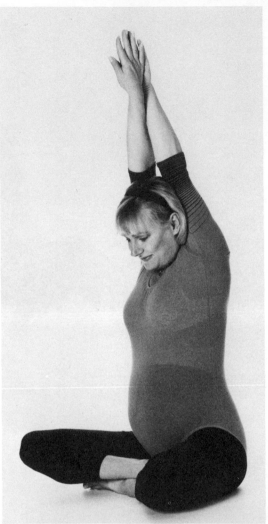

DAILY EXERCISE—DURING PREGNANCY

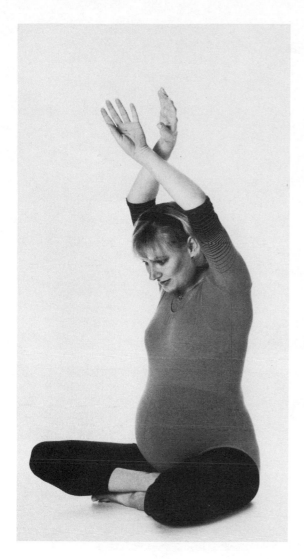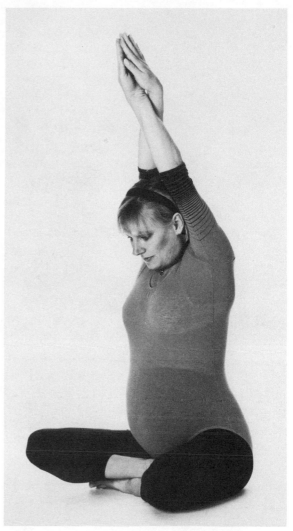

Upper Body Stretch

1. Sit upright, Indian-style, arms stretched forward, palms crossed and touching.
2. Lift arms high over your head, reach fingertips to ceiling, drop head forward—stretch.
3. Drop arms, cross the palms the opposite way, reach up, and stretch again.

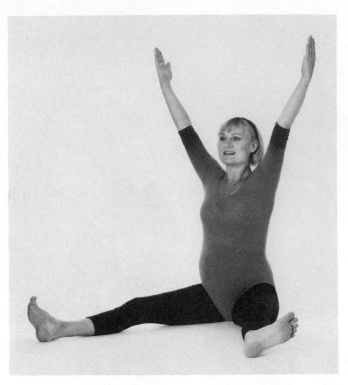

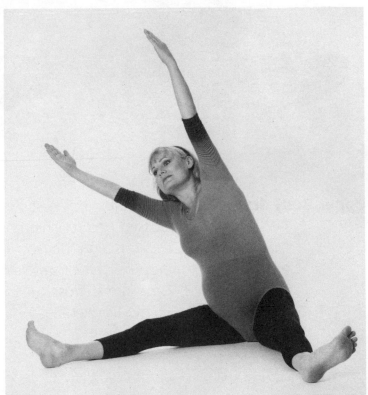

Spinal Stretch

1. Sit upright, legs comfortably apart, arms stretched upward, pull yourself out of your ribs as much as possible and stretch arms behind your ears.
2. Side lift, reach up and out diagonally toward the ceiling.
3. Spiral to right, reaching arms parallel to floor.

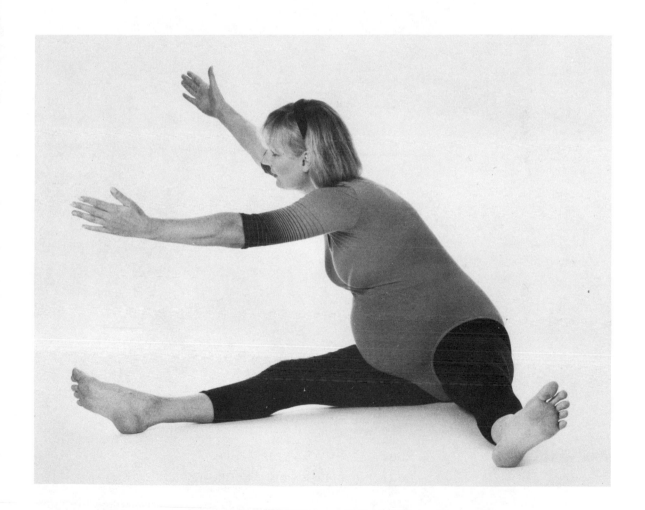

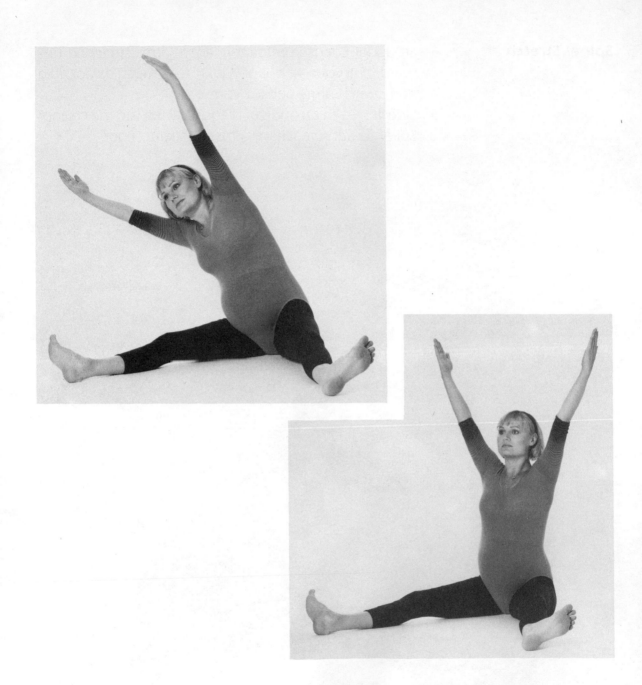

4. Return to the diagonal reach.
5. Return to first position. Repeat to left side.

DAILY EXERCISE—DURING PREGNANCY

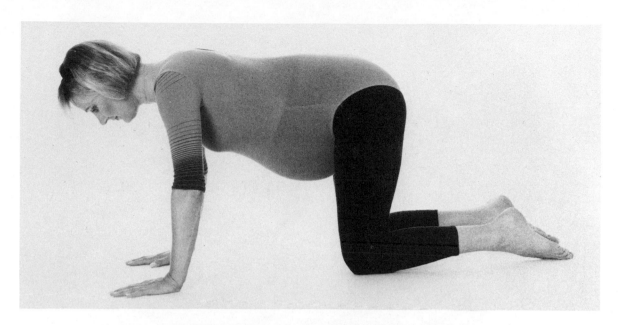

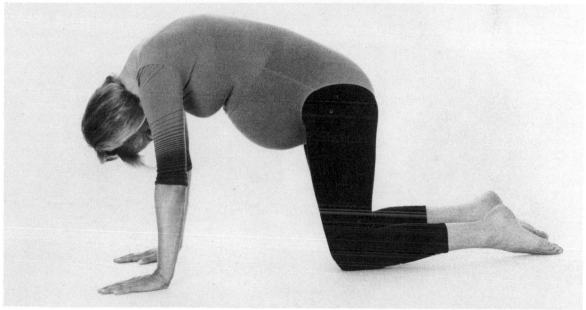

The Cat
with Variations

1. Start on all fours.
2. Curve spine toward ceiling.

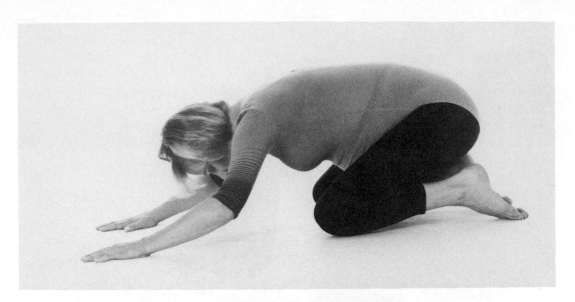

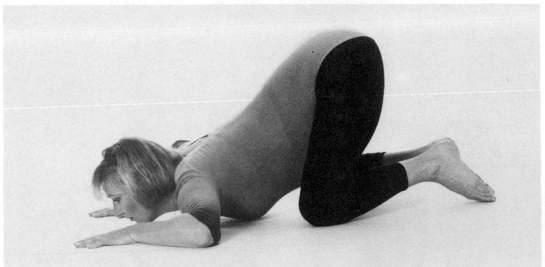

3. Sit back on heels.
4. Slide chest forward on floor and lift sitbones toward ceiling.
5. Straighten arms as chest reaches forward.
6. Arch or curve spine again toward ceiling.

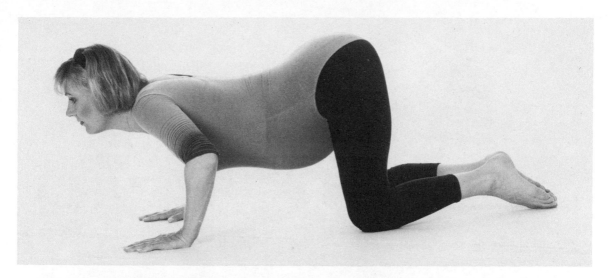

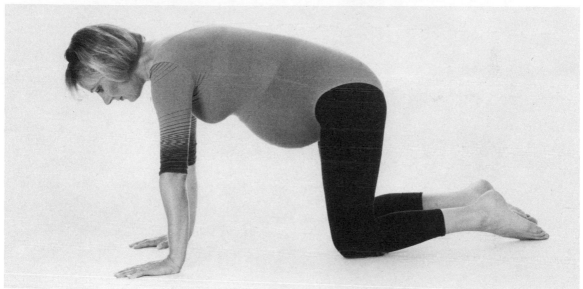

DAILY EXERCISE—DURING PREGNANCY

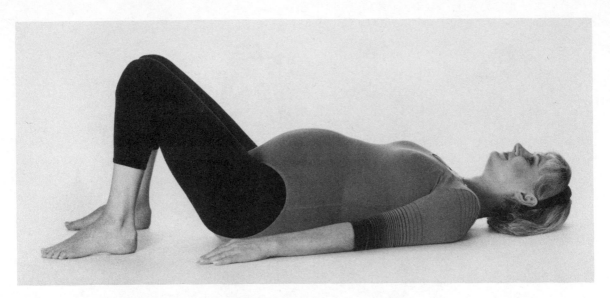

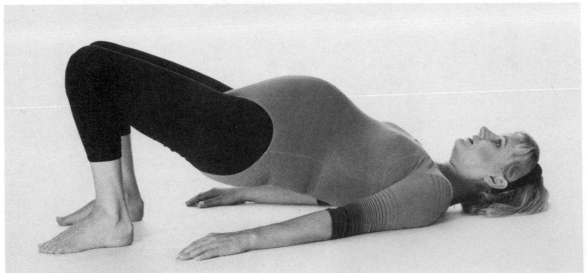

DAILY EXERCISE—DURING PREGNANCY

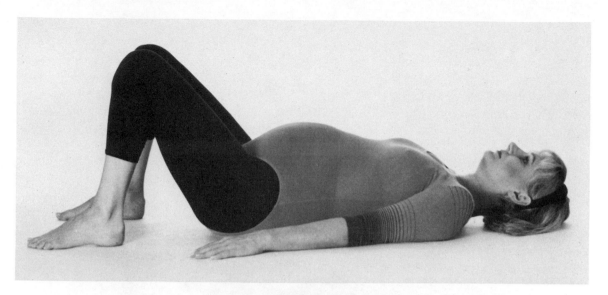

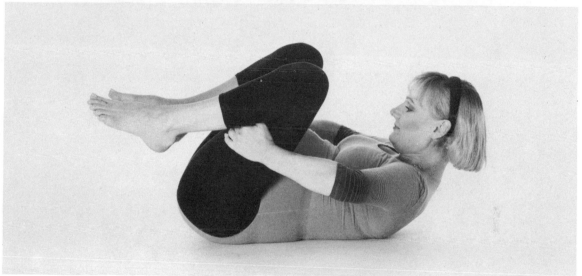

**The Bridge
with Variations**

1. Lie on back with knees bent.
2. Lift buttocks off floor, vertebra by vertebra.
3. Roll back, vertebra by vertebra.
4. Hold on to thighs—pull knees toward head and bring head forward toward knees.

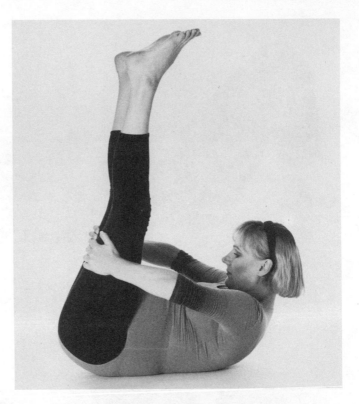

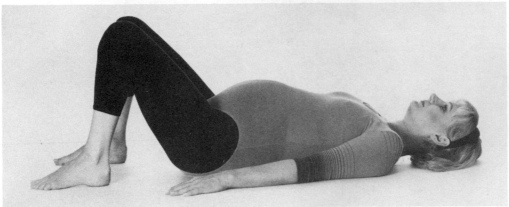

5. Stretch legs toward ceiling.
6. Return to first position and bend knees. Your back should be flat on the floor.

DAILY EXERCISE—DURING PREGNANCY

Spinal Roll

1. Stand—feet parallel, hip-width apart, arms reaching toward ceiling.
2. Bend forward from hips with straight back, fingers reaching forward.

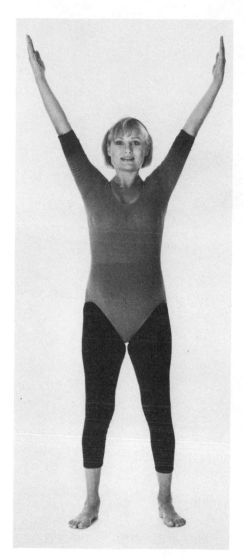

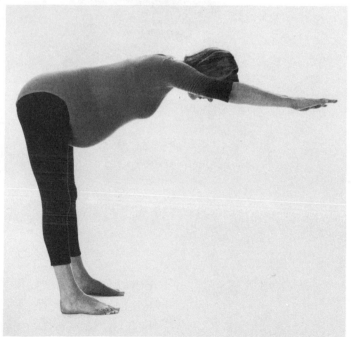

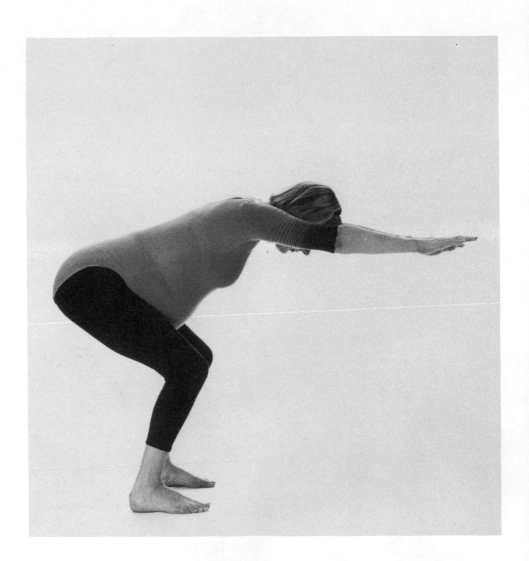

3. Bend knees, keep legs parallel and arms extended.
4. Relax upper body, let arms drop.
5. Roll up slowly, vertebra by vertebra.

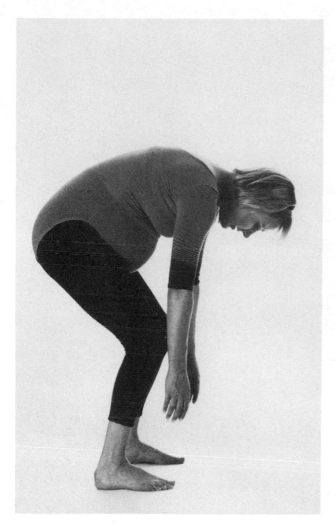
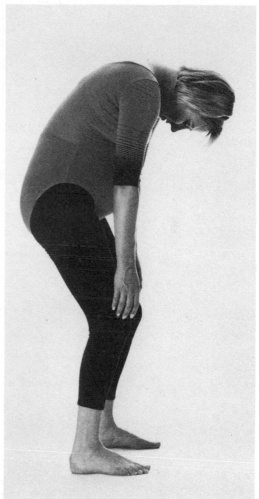

DAILY EXERCISE—DURING PREGNANCY

THE POSTPARTUM PERIOD–AT THE HOSPITAL

Mary gave birth to a little boy. Christopher weighed 8½ pounds; he was 21 inches tall. Her labor lasted three and a half hours, which was considerably shorter than her first labor, and she was fully able to participate, as she and Tom were well trained in the Lamaze method of childbirth. Mary felt a little fatigued, but one day after she had given birth she was ready to start a well-moderated exercise routine in the hospital.

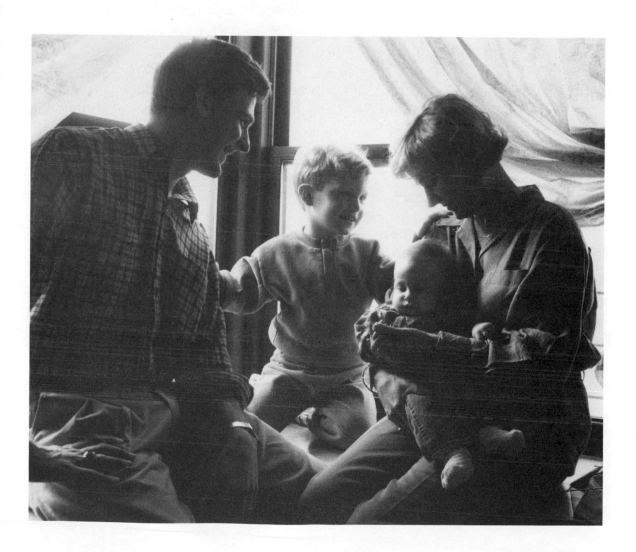

THE FIRST DAY POSTPARTUM

The very first thing Mary did, almost immediately after she settled in her room at the hospital, was to turn over on her stomach, putting a pillow under her belly so that she would not put any pressure on her breasts. She relaxed in this position for a good half hour the first day, and then every day for at least a half hour or more, reading, resting, or sleeping. It was the greatest luxury to her: being able to lie flat on her belly again after months and months of not being able to do so. This position helps involute the uterus—that is, make it go back to its original size.

Lying on Stomach

Before getting up or rolling over on her back again, Mary tightens her whole body, her back muscles, her abdominal muscles, and her legs. She holds her body tight and tense to the count of six, then relaxes. She repeats the tightening of back, abdomen, and legs, counts to six, and relaxes again.

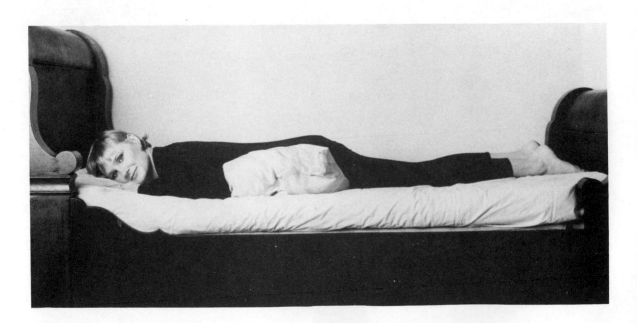

SECOND DAY POSTPARTUM

Mary has been up and about. She has been to the bathroom; she has had a shower, and she feels good, though a little achy all over. She has been doing her Kegel exercises since the day before. She tightens her pelvic floor, holds it tight, and relaxes it again. She tries to do this as often as thirty times a day, whenever she thinks of it. It is not easy for Mary to exercise her pelvic floor muscles, as the whole area still feels very sore. During her delivery, her doctor performed an episiotomy. This small incision in the area between the anus and the vagina is done shortly before the baby's head emerges, to speed the delivery of the baby's head and perhaps prevent tearing.

Exercising the pelvic floor area speeds up the healing process. Contraction and relaxation of the area increase new blood supply and at the same time squeeze out old blood.

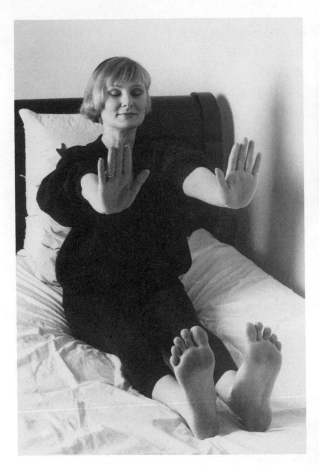 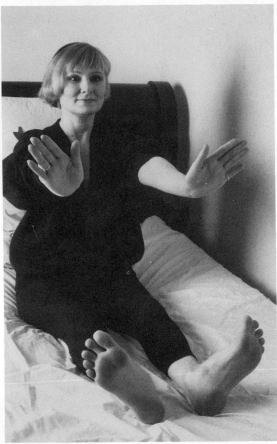

Hands, Wrists, and Feet

Mary is sitting up in bed. She stretches her arms forward to shoulder level, extends her wrists upward, and flexes her feet. As she inhales, she rotates both hands and feet out and down. As she exhales, she completes the circle with both hands and feet, rotating them in and down and back to the original position. She repeats this exercise ten times.

Working with hands, wrists, and feet will not only improve the circulation but will insure good mobility in the joints.

84

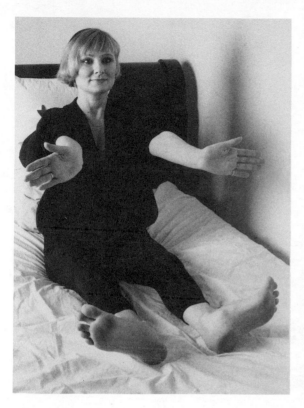

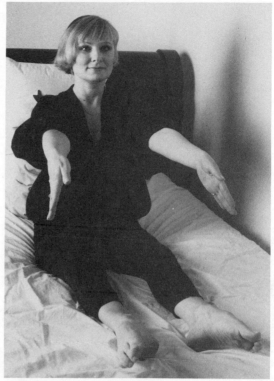

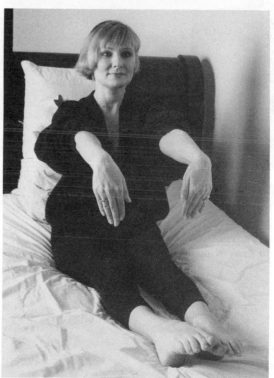

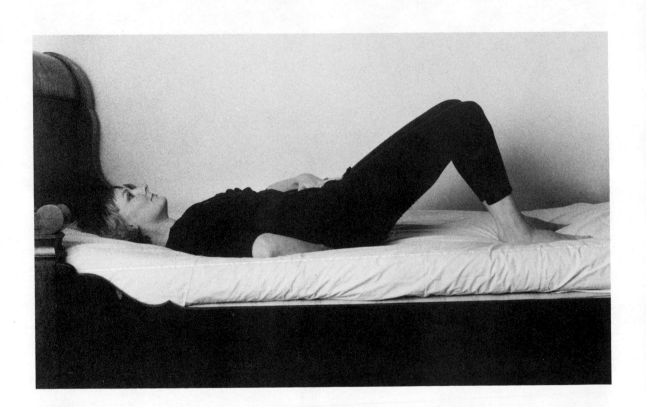

**Hug and Lift—
Pelvic Tilt**

Mary is lying on her bed. She bends her legs, her feet resting firmly on the bed. She inhales, and as she exhales, she tightens her abdominal muscles and flattens her back against the bed. As she inhales, she releases her back and abdomen. Then, as she is exhaling again, she tightens her belly and flattens her back. Mary repeats this exercise with breathing six times.

THIRD DAY POSTPARTUM

The typical hospital stay after delivery is much shorter these days than it used to be. Mary was sent home on day three. She is continuing her exercises regularly, even taking her afternoon nap resting on her belly. She continues the exercise in which she tightens her stomach, her back, her legs, counts to six, and releases all the tension in her body (page 82). She repeats this six times. She always remembers to do her Kegel exercises, and she enjoys the pelvic tilt (page 86). Next she sits up, stretches, and closes her fingers into a tight fist. She also rotates her hands and feet in both directions, and repeats this exercise six times.

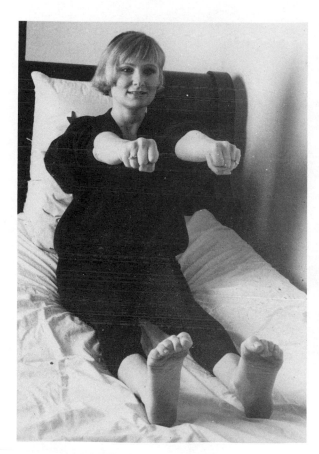 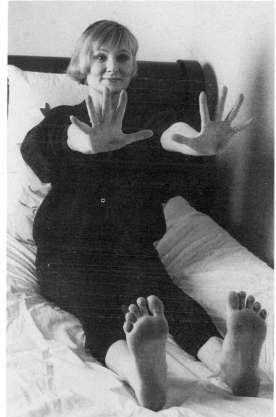

On the third day after the baby's birth, Mary can begin a new exercise.

Spinal Stretch

1. Sit cross-legged. Inhale, arms behind your head, arch upper back, look at ceiling. Exhale, bend your head forward, and push your nose into your chest. Lift your head, inhale, exhale, and lower your head. Let your elbows drop down. Repeat six times, dropping your head as you exhale. Inhale as you stretch up, elbows wide.

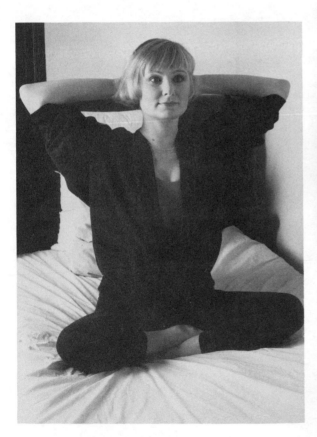 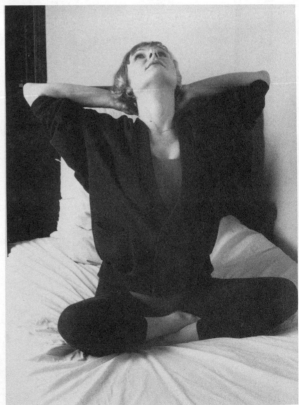

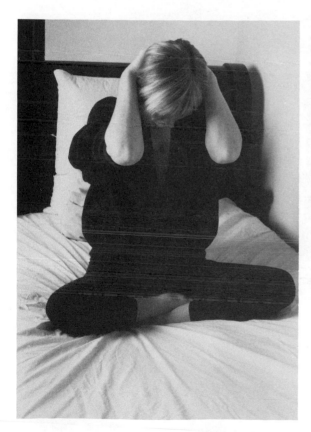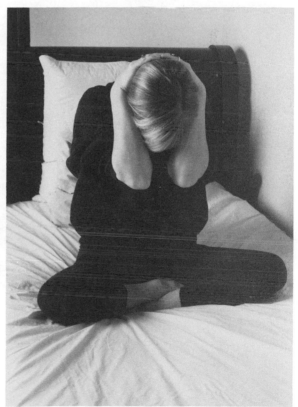

THE POSTPARTUM PERIOD—AT THE HOSPITAL

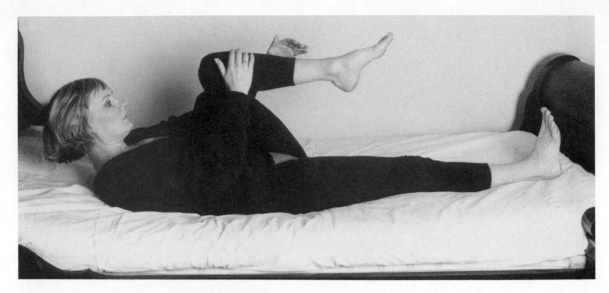

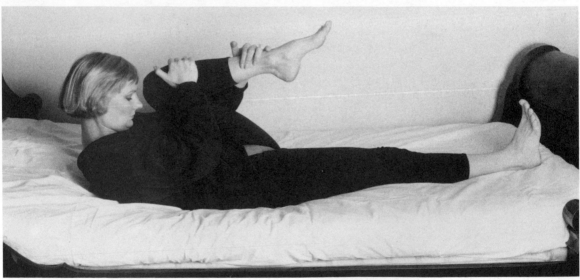

2. Lie down. Bend left knee up, with the left hand on your ankle, right hand on knee. Bend knee and head toward each other as you exhale. Return leg to rest on bed, repeat lifting head and leg toward each other six times.

3. Knee drop. Lie on your back, bend knees, feet hip-width apart. Inhale, then exhale and bend both knees to the right, inhale and bring both knees back to upright position. Keep shoulders flat on bed. Repeat with breathing to left. Repeat three times each side.

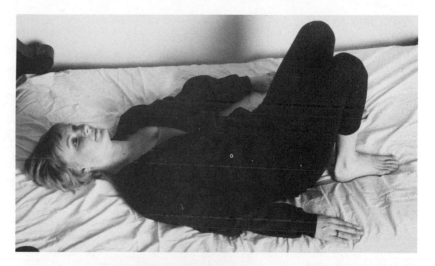

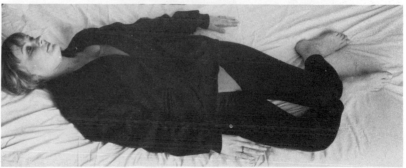

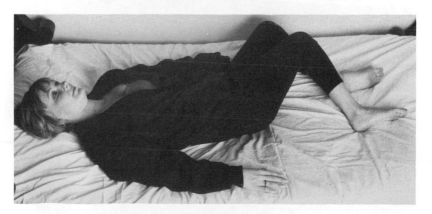

THE DAILY
EXERCISE ROUTINE
—POSTPARTUM

These exercises are particularly useful for three to six months postpartum. They can also serve as a basis for a general exercise routine.

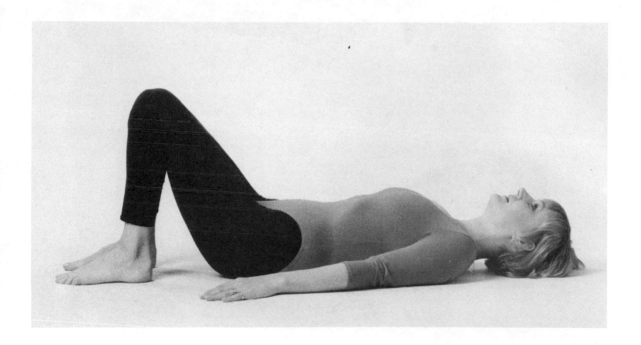

The Bridge   1. Lie on your back, knees bent, feet firmly on the ground.

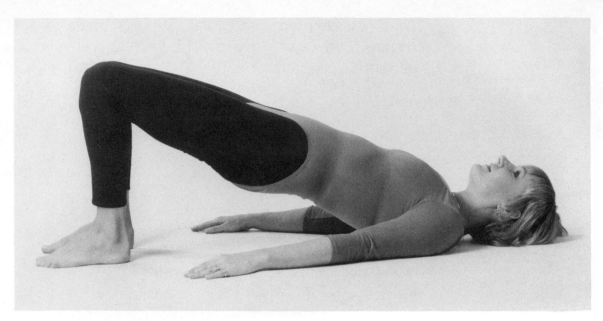

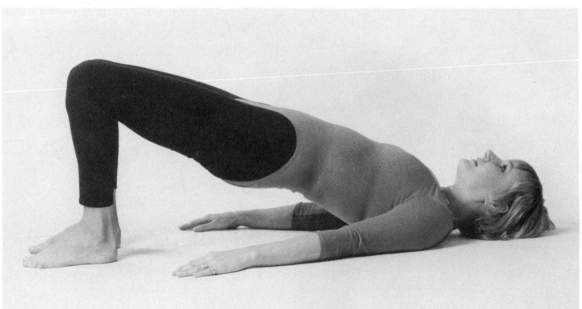

2. Inhale, then exhale and lift your pelvis up, vertebra by vertebra—inhale.

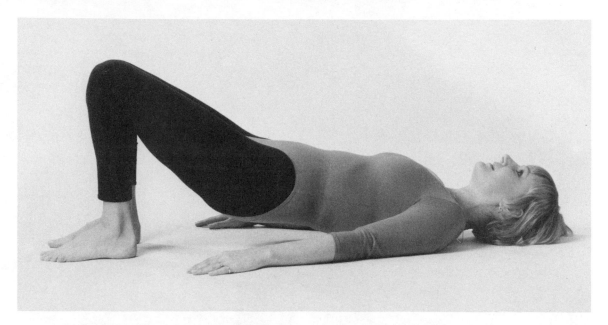

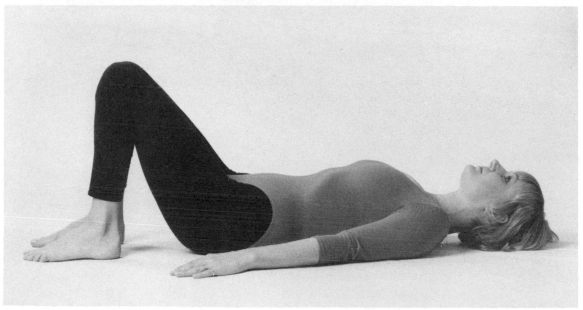

3. Exhale and lower your back slowly, vertebra by vertebra.

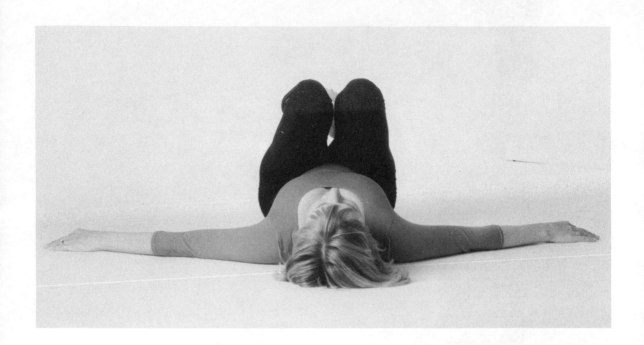

Hip Rotation

1. Lie on your back, knees bent and feet off the floor.
2. Inhale, then exhale and lower knees to your left. Extend legs. Arms are stretched out at right angles, keep shoulders on the floor.

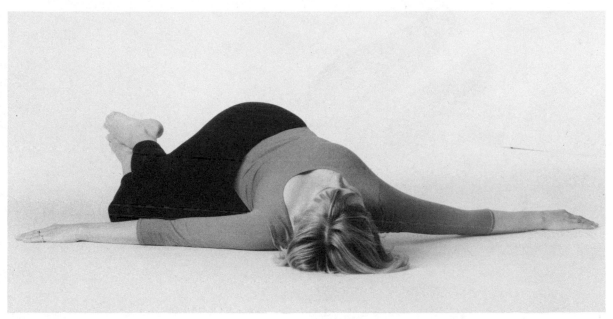

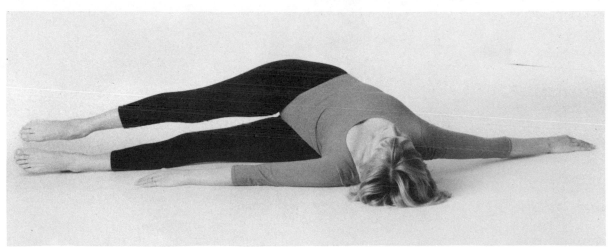

3. Inhale. Then exhale, bend legs, and bring both knees back to center.
4. Repeat with breathing to the right. Do the exercise three times to each side.

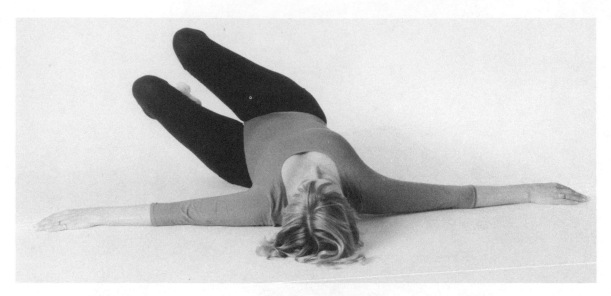

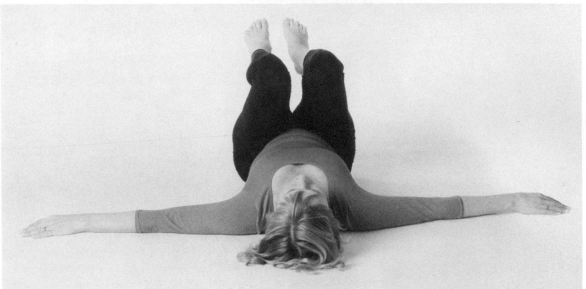

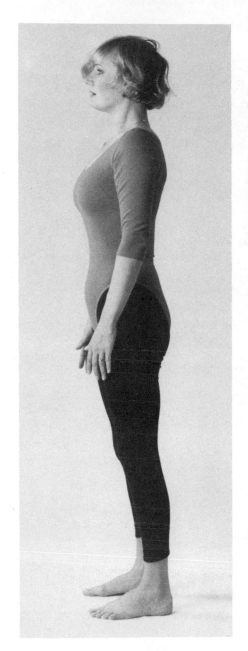 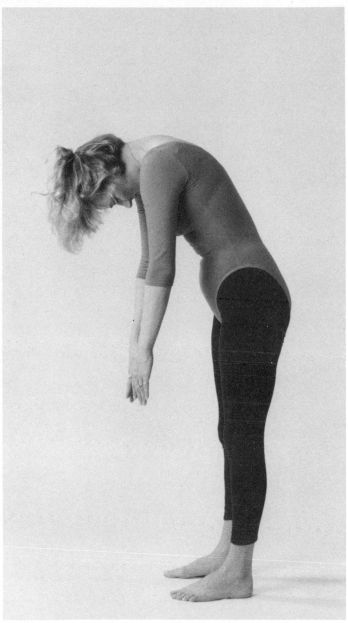

**Roll Down
and Relax**

1. Stand erect, feet firmly on ground, hip-width apart.
2. Inhale, then exhale and slowly lower your back.

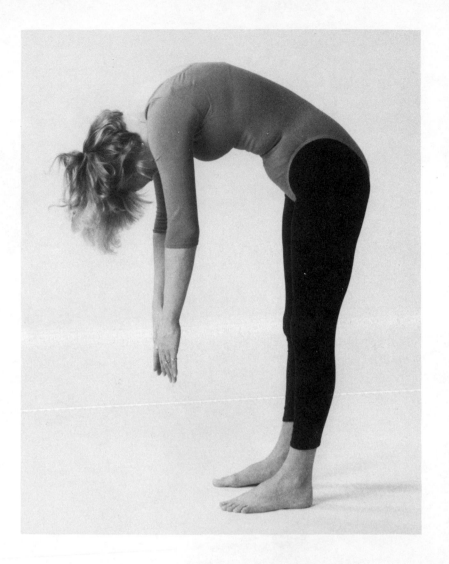

3. When you are down, place your right hand on your
   left shoulder and your left hand on your right shoulder.
4. Hang relaxed and continue breathing slowly as long
   as it is comfortable.
5. Roll up slowly, vertebra by vertebra.
   This exercise will strengthen your oblique abdominals
and help get your body into good shape.

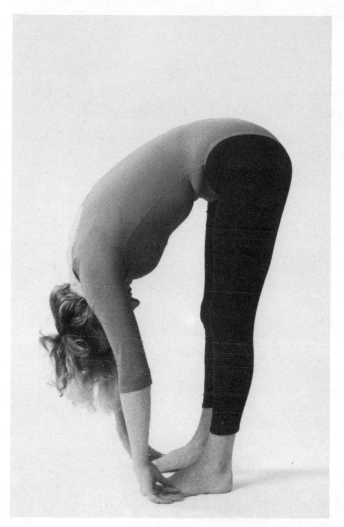
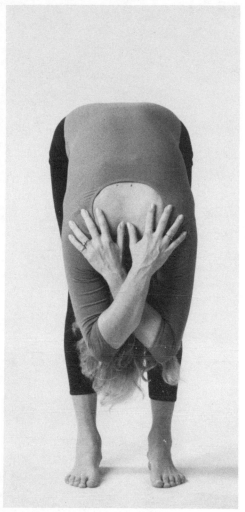

Rollbacks

This is quite a strenuous exercise, but it's an excellent way to build up your abdominal muscles.

1. Sit with your legs bent and feet firmly on the ground.
2. Inhale, exhale, and then lean back with your arms stretched forward to an angle of 60–65 degrees.
3. Inhale again and come back to a straight sitting position as you exhale.

Repeat this exercise five times.

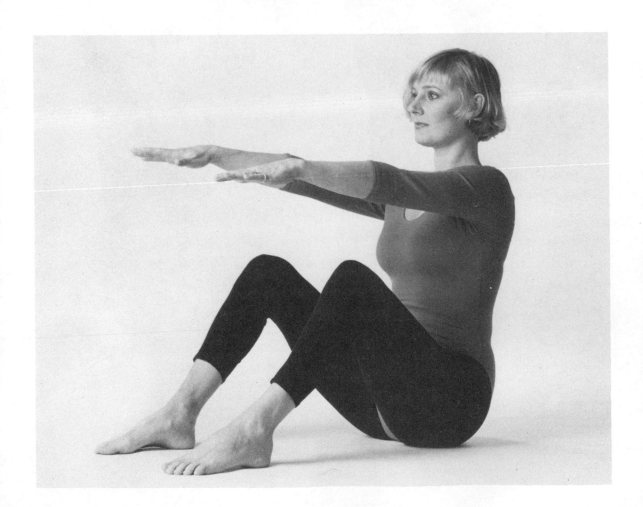

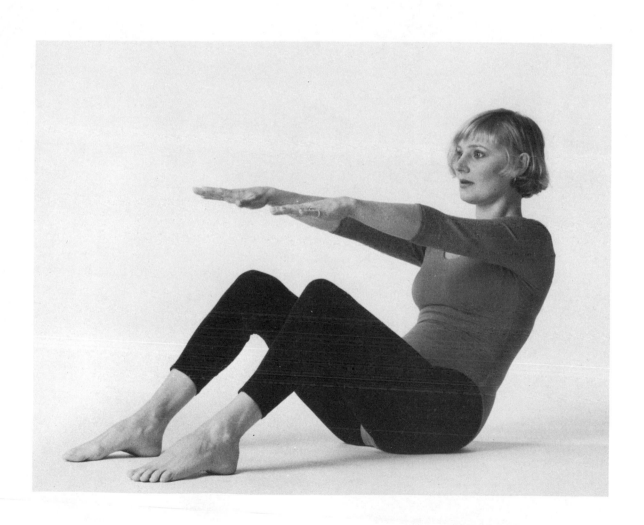

DAILY EXERCISE—POSTPARTUM

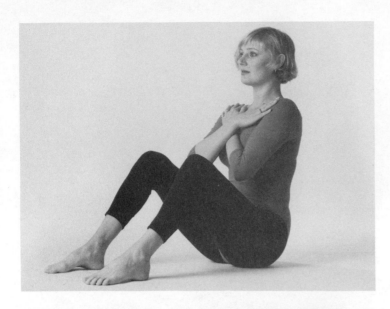

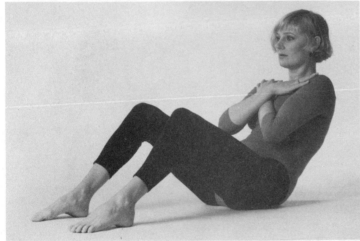

Here are two variations:

A.

1. Instead of stretching your arms forward, fold your arms over your chest.
2. Inhale, then exhale and lean back.
3. Inhale, and exhale as you straighten out again.

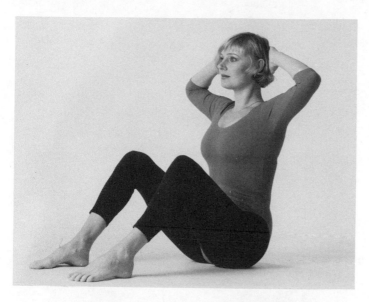

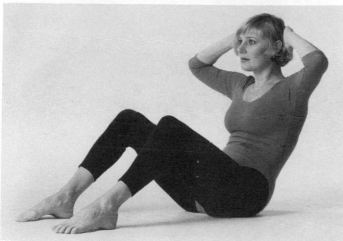

B.

1. Place your hands behind your head.
2. Inhale, then exhale and lean back.
3. Inhale, then exhale and come back to a straight sitting position.

Try to work up to doing each variation five times.

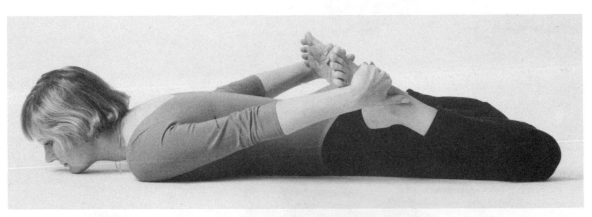

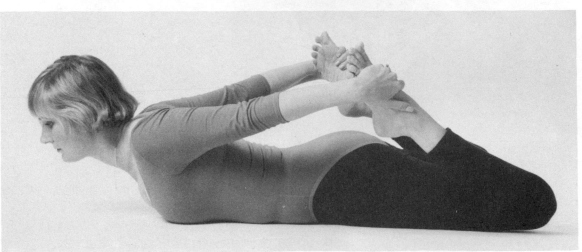

DAILY EXERCISE—POSTPARTUM

The Bow

This exercise will strengthen your back muscles and at the same time give your abdominals a good massage.

1. Lie on your belly and bend your knees. Hold on to your feet.
2. Inhale, exhale, and pull up your chest and legs.
3. Continue to breathe as you seesaw back and forth on your belly. Try to lift your thighs off the floor. This gives your thighs an excellent stretch.

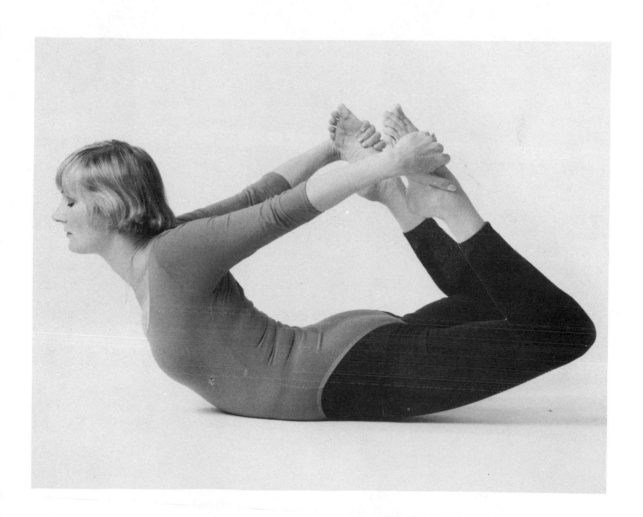

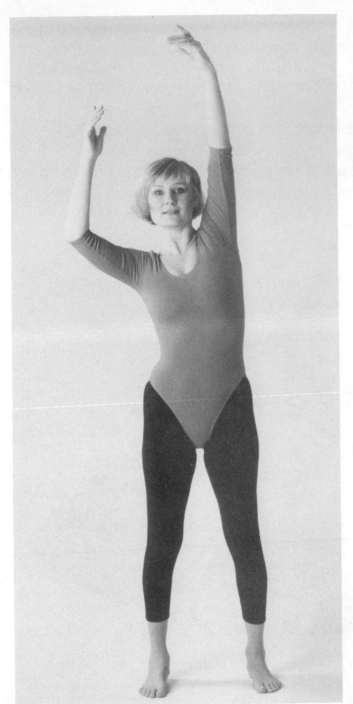

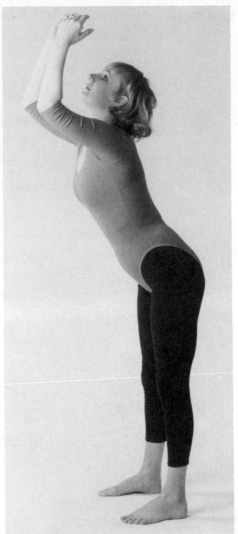

DAILY EXERCISE—POSTPARTUM

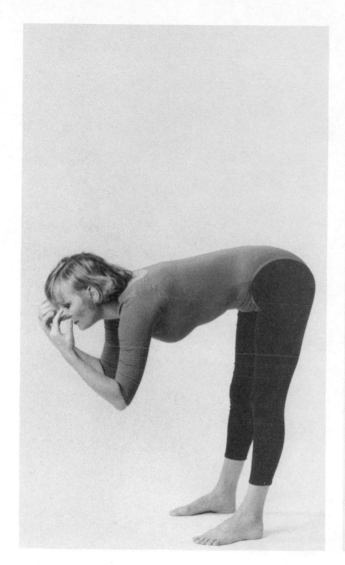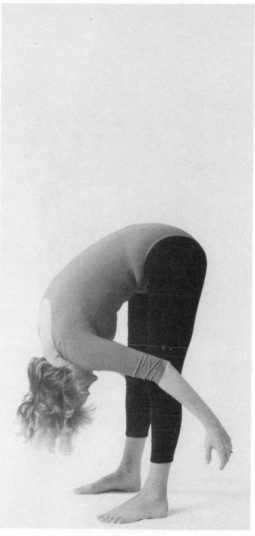

Stretch and Swing Your Body

This is one of my favorite exercises. You will find that it feels good to stretch your whole body and swing your back down and up for mobility.

1. Stand straight and reach arms toward the ceiling.
2. Swing your arms forward and down as you bend your back.

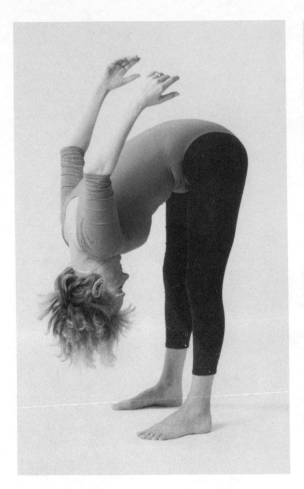 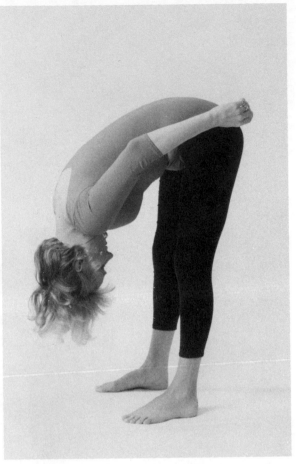

3. Swing your arms forward and up again and let your arms pull you upright again.

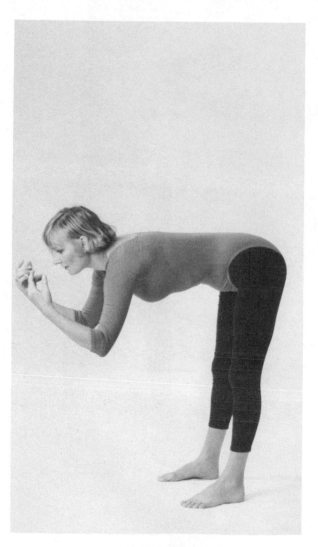 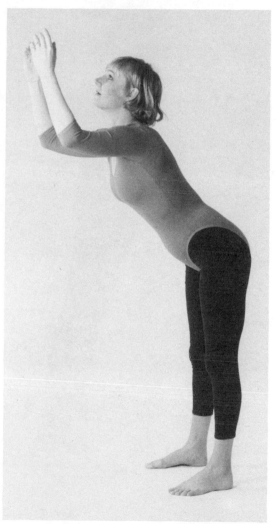

DAILY EXERCISE—POSTPARTUM

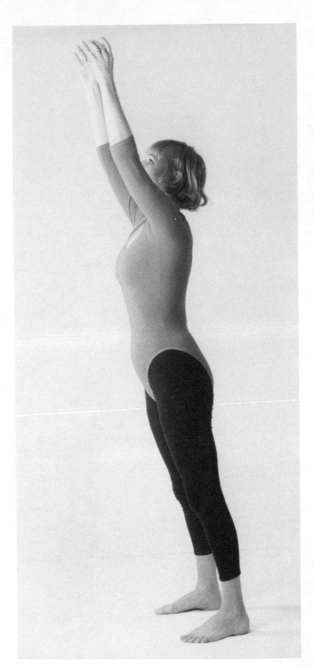
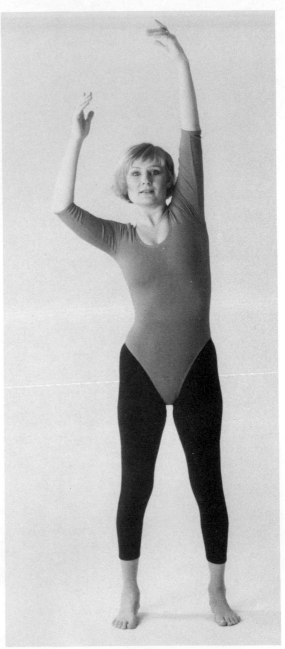

4. Swing down and up at least six times.

DAILY EXERCISE—POSTPARTUM

The Seesaw with Christopher

This exercise is mainly for fun. Your baby will love being rocked.

1. Lie on your back, bend your knees with thighs touching, feet off the floor.
2. Put the baby on your shins and support him well with your hands.
3. Inhale, then exhale and stretch legs up to a 35 degree angle. Slowly lower your legs as you inhale again, exhale, and stretch legs up again. Let the baby's weight pull your legs down. Repeat this exercise, stretching and bending your legs, five to eight times.

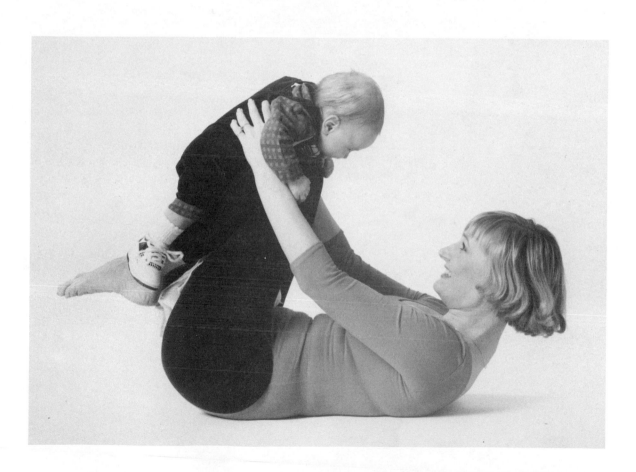

EPILOGUE

Working on a book is generally hard work, frustrating, lonely, and often satisfactory only in retrospect. But working on this book was almost always enjoyable, hardly ever lonely, full of fun and a great deal of laughter. I want to thank Mary and Tom and young Matthew for their wonderful cooperation, their professionalism, and even their enthusiasm about our project. In fact, we got so involved with the photographs that we tended to forget the time and even occasionally overtaxed Mary.

Jill Strickman, our photographer, was always patient with all of us, joining in the fun and often trying out some of the exercises herself. Jamie Stiller, our choreographer, helped with her knowledge and years of experience of pre- and postnatal exercises. Elisabeth Dyssegaard, my editor, was always there, helping, encouraging, and supervising. What a great team we had!

As a childbirth educator, I'm lucky to have the chance to share a few weeks of a couple's life during their pregnancy and some weeks or months after the birth. Mary and Tom were very special in sharing this period in their lives not only with me and the photographer but with all of you who will use this book.